MORE PRA...

Guns A' Blazing

"*Guns A' Blazing* is an interesting mix of personal experiences and pertinent aspects of special education law that will be helpful for new as well as experienced parents to special education. This book is an easy-to-read and easy-to-understand manual to guide parents and teachers along the maze of rules, standards, and hopes for children and students with autism spectrum disorders. *Guns A' Blazing* tackles difficult situations such as lunch time and recess at school, and preparing children for adulthood."

– Kirby Lentz, Ed.D., President/CEO, Chileda, La Crosse, Wisconsin, and Author of *Hopes and Dreams: An IEP Guide for Parents of Children with Autism Spectrum Disorders*

"What a wonderful book! Based on the lived experiences of the author, his wife, their son, and the professionals with whom they have worked, this book provides much insight into the 'schooling' process for a child with Asperger Syndrome (AS). It highlights the challenges parents and professionals face when trying to provide effective educational experiences for a student with AS, sharing what Cohen and his wife have learned about working effectively with school personnel. While it is an excellent book for parents of children with AS, we plan to use it as a required readings book in our graduate course, Methods for Students with Asperger's Syndrome."

– Marj Bock, Associate Professor and Director, Global Rural Autism Asperger Information Network

GUNS A' BLAZING

GUNS A' BLAZING

How Parents of Children on the Autism Spectrum and Schools Can Work Together – Without a Shot Being Fired

Jeffrey Cohen

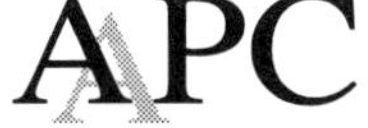

Autism Asperger Publishing Co.
P.O. Box 23173
Shawnee Mission, Kansas 66283-0173
www.asperger.net

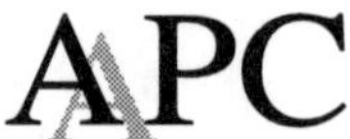

P.O. Box 23173
Shawnee Mission, Kansas 66283-0173
www.asperger.net

PUBLISHER'S CATALOGING-IN-PUBLICATION

Cohen, Jeffrey.

Guns a' blazing: how parents of children on the autism spectrum and schools can work together – without a shot being fired / Jeffrey Cohen. – lst ed. – Shawnee Mission, Kan.: Autism Asperger Pub. Co., 2006.

p. ; cm.

ISBN-1 3: 978-1-931282-86-4 (pbk.)
ISBN-10: 1-931282-86-2 (pbk.)
LCCN 2005935603
Summary: Teachers, administrators, professionals and many parents contribute ideas and offer advice on topics ranging from home schooling to transition plans to college.

1. Autistic children—Education. 2. Autism in children. 3. Asperger's syndrome – Patients – Education. 4. Learning disabled children – Education. 5. Parent-teacher relationships. I. Title.

LC4717.C64 2006 2005935603
371.94-dc22 0512

This book is designed in Adobe Caslon and Zebrawood.

Printed in the United States of America.

Dedication

This book is gratefully dedicated to all the public school teachers, administrators and experts who have helped my son through school, particularly Joyce Gregus, without whom I'm sure it wouldn't have been possible. Thanks to all of you for helping me keep my guns in their holsters.

Acknowledgments

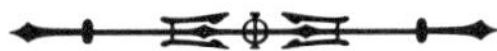

I can't adequately thank the people who really wrote this book: the parents, teachers, administrators, psychologists, social workers, educational consultants, speech and language experts, therapists and countless others who answered a plea for help with their time, their understanding and their stories. But especially, I wish to thank the children whose stories were told for allowing their parents and me to use them as illustrations and hopefully help those who will come next.

To the parents who took the time to sit down for an interview that inevitably lasted longer than I said it would, I could thank you for the next 215 pages, and it wouldn't be enough. Those of you who agreed to let me mention your names are listed below. Those of you who asked to remain anonymous are just as gratefully acknowledged.

To the professionals who answered my questions without taking offense, I applaud your ongoing efforts to help every child who passes into your lives. Please try to understand that the parents who come in with Guns A' Blazing are acting out of concern for their children, and not because they want to make your lives difficult. Thanks for your efforts.

Thanks also to my favorite editor, Kirsten McBride, to Keith Myles for giving me so much leeway, and to everyone whom I've met in traveling around to speak about Asperger Syndrome first, and autism spectrum disorders in general. I've never felt so welcome, and I appreciate it every time.

Parents: Lauren Agoratus (Family Voices), Debra Auslander, Bonnie Berginski, Theresa Berwieler, Maggie Bishop, Sandi Bongart, E. Jennifer Brown, Nancy Carey-Richardson, Kristine Chronheim, Patti Conard, Ann Creswell, Karen Dawson, Karen Donnelly, Karen Douglass, Julie Esris, Etho Foxhill, Jodi Fugl, Ruth J. Henderson, Diane Hollister, Earl and Martha Hyde, Joan Johnson (PTI Nebraska), Lorey Leddy, Michelle Matathia, Susan Matson, Michele Maynard, Debra Noonan-Elber, Sharie Ostrowski, Nicole S. Peters, Bernice Polinsky, Suzanne Reek, Jim Rodenhiser, Jon Rowland, Karen Salomon, Barbara Sidrer, Sharon Solar, Carol Solon, Paula Stark, Kim Szeremeta, Elly Tucker, Amy Van Hoover, Didi Zaryczny (Commonwealth Autism).

Professionals: Ellyn Atherton, Ira Fingles, Steve Rosen, the kind people of COSAC, Greg Moorehead of Rutgers University, and many others who asked not to be named, or whom I ended up not quoting, but using their information for background. I appreciate your time and your dedication. Please, don't stop.

Table of Contents

Introduction

HOLSTER THAT WEAPON, SOLDIER!

"Look, we know our son can be an enormous pain in the butt."

The atmosphere around the conference table visibly relaxed. The teachers, administrators, psychologist, social worker and special education instructor all sat back in their chairs, smiling with relief. You could practically hear each one sigh internally.

The annual IEP (Individualized Education Program) meeting about our son Joshua, then a 9-year-old with Asperger Syndrome (AS), was going to be a lot easier now. My wife and I, by admitting that our son wasn't a perfect student, had opened the door for an honest discussion, and we'd alleviated the school system's fears that we'd expect the moon when all they could offer was a succession of asteroids.

And let's face it: Especially in those days, Josh – who is 15 years old and a high school freshman at this writing – could be a huge pain. His legendarily short temper got him into arguments with other students and teachers, fights he didn't have a hope of winning. He could be obstinate and stubborn, could complain about virtually any aspect of the school day and could, in class, be counted on to pay attention and participate – whenever he felt like it. Otherwise, there was a good deal of staring out the window. And flapping of hands. And singing, sometimes quietly, to himself.

We had entered the meeting a little unsure of ourselves. While it was not Josh's first IEP meeting, it was the first one in his new school (our system has primary, elementary, middle and high schools, and this was the step from primary to elementary). We didn't know the principal or teachers as well as we might, and the paraprofessional who was Josh's class aide was new to us. She has since been with him for seven years and counting – a major coup.

As parents, we knew what we needed to accomplish at this meeting. We wanted to make sure Josh's teacher for the coming year would we one who would understand his unique needs and be able to deal with them. (There was, it should be noted, one teacher we had been warned to avoid at all costs.) We wanted to make sure his aide stayed with him. We wanted assurances that he could type assignments into a computer when the torturous process of writing longhand became too much for him to handle. And we wanted Josh to have a "safe room" where he could excuse himself from class and cool down when it was necessary.

The school system, having dealt with Asperger parents for only a few years (this was 1998, only four years after AS was listed in the DSM IV [*Diagnostic and Statistical Manual of Mental Disorders*] as a diagnosis), wasn't sure how reasonable – or unreasonable – we were prepared to be. Some parents, we were told later, had asked for lunch periods away from all other children and with outside food brought in, advance looks at tests so parents could "quiz" the child ahead of time, a permanent excuse from physical education and separate tutors in each subject, even when the child's grades were all A's and B's.

In other words, they didn't know what to expect from us, and we didn't know what to expect from them. Given that set of circumstances, it was understandable that both sides were a little leery.

So, I had chosen to break the ice with the acknowledgment that there were times when Josh drove me crazy, too.

The laughter that followed my statement was more a testament to the relief evident in the room than the level of humor.

When parents are reasonable and realistic about their children, it's much easier for school systems to be the same.

My friend Lori Shery, co-founder of ASPEN, the Asperger Syndrome Education Network (www.aspennj.org), says that a lot of Asperger Parents (and parents throughout the autism spectrum) enter any encounter with their school systems by assuming they are going to be misled, patronized, condescended to and otherwise swindled out of the services their children legitimately need to get through the school year. So they walk in with that attitude practically tattooed on their foreheads, breathing fire and acting defensive before there's anything to defend. Lori calls it "going in with Guns A' Blazing." It's an understandable response, since many school systems, particularly public school systems strapped for funding, indeed try to withhold as many services as possible to save on the bottom line.

But most educators, from classroom teachers up to superintendents, are dedicated to doing all they can to help each child, particularly those with special needs. They really want to deliver whatever services will help our children achieve all they can, but they are hamstrung by limitations imposed by budgets, state regulations and the needs of an increasing number of special needs students. In New Jersey, where I live, the diagnoses of AS and autism have skyrocketed over the past 10 years, and that means more of a strain on school budgets and more of a strain on the professionals who administer them and teach our children. The same is true in most other places across the country.

That's not meant to be an excuse for shoddy work or imperious professionals who believe autism and AS are a myth, that we as parents are being either too easy on our children or overparenting them to the point that we expect more than they deserve. Those points of view are absurd and unreasonable. I'm trying to explain why school officials, from teachers on up, are somewhat leery of autism spectrum parents.

When our guns are a' blazing, we can sometimes be a little scary.

After I had told the members of the IEP meeting that our son wasn't perfect – or more specifically, that we knew our son wasn't perfect – there was a better sense of cooperation around the table. We knew what we were here to do, who we were here to help, and the possibility of competition gave way to one of working toward a common goal.

It was a calculated move. I wanted to convey very clearly that we weren't expecting miracles, but that we were expecting help, and that we understood it was needed. The school officials wanted my wife and me to know that they were anxious to give our son the help he needed, but that they couldn't deal with someone who thought everything that went wrong was the school's fault. With one sentence, I had managed to wipe that impression away.

However, it's important to know when guns should be a' blazing. There are times when schools, teachers and administrators really are shirking their responsibility, when they really don't understand, or don't want to understand, what AS and HFA (high-functioning autism) mean and how they affect our children, and at those times, it's necessary to use every possible tool to obtain what our children need.

But it's never the best thing to do first.

It's important to give school administrators and teachers the chance to show you they're interested, capable and concerned before you decide they're indifferent, incompetent and impatient. Give them the benefit of the doubt, even if you've consulted with other parents of children with special needs in the district and been told the system is not the best on such issues. Listen to the horror stories other parents tell you, but factor in what you know about the parents' expectations. Were they realistic? Are the parents you're consulting the type who demand more than they should, who place unreasonable demands on the system? Would they be dissatisfied even if the school gave them everything they wanted?

In this book, you'll hear the horror stories. Some children on the spectrum really have been treated poorly, and some school systems – both public and private – have forced parents into court over placement and services for children who desperately needed them. Some teachers have accused parents of lying about their children's needs. Some administrators have flat-out denied that reported incidents between spectrum children and teachers have occurred, even when there were witnesses.

These are the times when it seems you should go in with Guns A' Blazing, figuratively speaking. These are the times that send some parents to professional advocates for help at IEP meetings. They add to the practices of attorneys who specialize in disability law. And in some cases, they convince parents that the only workable way to educate their children is by schooling them at home. All those cases will be examined in this book.

But there are other stories, too. The ones where parents and teachers work together to come up with reasonable solutions. The ones that begin as horror stories and conclude with almost fairy tale endings. The ones that give us hope to keep going back until our children get the kind of attention and services they need, to help them learn the things they need to learn, and do so without a severe disadvantage before they begin.

None of this is meant to advocate, or dismiss, any of the solutions reached. Home schooling works for some people; for others, it doesn't. Inclusion with an aide is the best solution we've found for our son, but some parents might consider inclusion with neurotypical children too difficult, or the one-on-one aide too obtrusive. It doesn't mean these plans are wrong; it means they're wrong for a given child at least in the parents' estimation. Your job is to sift through all the information and then make an informed decision for your child, based on the data, your knowledge of your child and your school, and your own feelings. This book will not tell you what to do. It is here to lay out the options, tell you what the advantages and pitfalls of each might be and, I hope, give you enough information to make up your own mind.

It will not be based only on my experience, luckily for you. Many wonderful parents of children on the autism spectrum volunteered (usually with great enthusiasm) to tell their stories, often in long telephone interviews during busy days when they easily could have opted to do something else. (Many of the interviews were conducted in and around the holiday season of 2004, for many parents the busiest time of year when children are home and there are many family obligations to meet.) They are from states in every part of the country, and some are from countries around the world – fortunately, they all spoke English, or I'd have been in a very difficult situation indeed!

I've also spoken to teachers, school administrators, parent advocates, lawyers and doctors. I can already hear the angry parents out there complaining about "taking their side." I learned long ago that there are three sides to every story – yours, theirs and the truth – and this is no exception. By better understanding how schools and their personnel operate, what their concerns might be and why they might not give you the answer you want right away, maybe it'll be easier to determine what can be done, what to ask for and how to ask.

Going into a school, as a parent, is not all that different from going in when you're a child. You're still nervous about being summoned to the principal's office, and it's a little intimidating to deal with people who have a very secure grip (it seems) on what can and can't be done, and then ask for something else. There's no reason to be afraid. As my father used to say to me, "the worst they can do is say no."

And that's when the hard-working parent gets busy compiling data, explaining procedures and reasons, talking to anyone who will listen, determining options and executing plans. Because "no" is just the beginning in some stories.

Going in with Guns A' Blazing on the first visit isn't the way to go. At least wait until they say no.

And remember, once you've read this book, the experiences and wisdom of literally hundreds of people will be with you. You're not going in alone.

Chapter One

GUNS A' BLAZING

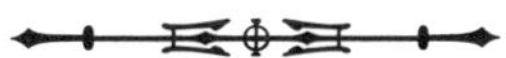

Nothing gets me angrier than someone who treats my son Josh like a Poor Afflicted Child (PAC), someone worthy of pity, but not respect. The people who take my hand tenderly and ask in their best "concerned" voice, "so how is Josh" are the ones most likely to be given a sarcastic response. If they don't accept, "He's fine, and how are you?" but try even harder to show me how "tolerant" they are of the PAC, I will not be held responsible for my actions.

So understand that when I attended my first IEP meeting, when Josh was in kindergarten, I was ready to be treated like the parent of a PAC. I'd been treated that way by neighbors, (distant) family members and even some psychologists and physicians since he was 18 months old. One doctor had informed us in no uncertain terms that our son would always be "eccentric." I couldn't resist telling him that we couldn't afford "eccentric;" we were only middle-class parents. The best we could do was "neurotic." He'd have to work harder. For my trouble, I was given a glance that indicated he knew now where the eccentricity might have originated.

I entered that first IEP meeting, to plan for Josh's transition into first grade, with a certain amount of attitude. I knew he had a diagnosis of Asperger Syndrome, and I had done enough research to understand what that meant, but my wife and I were determined not to treat Josh like a PAC. He had challenges, and we'd do our best to help him meet them. If he needed special help, we were there to be sure he'd get it.

When the meeting began, and the first suggestion was that Joshua not go immediately into first grade the following year, the hair on the back of my neck began to stand up. This was exactly the kind of condescending, patronizing suggestion I'd assumed I'd hear – they were telling me my son wasn't smart enough for first grade, yet I knew he had no issues with academics. They just didn't understand what Asperger Syndrome was, I figured (keep in mind that this was 1995, and nobody knew what Asperger Syndrome was, really).

I was about to protest, but I made a choice. This was the beginning, I believed, of what was to be a long road, and to get off on the wrong foot could be a terrible miscalculation. So I held my comments for the moment, and decided to just listen.

Aside from marrying Josh's mother, that was the best choice I've ever made.

The school system's speech and language therapist, who would become the fiercest and most loyal advocate my son had in the school system, explained that the Child Study Team felt the most appropriate option for Josh was a year in a program they called "Transitional Primary." They understood that he had no academic issues, and weren't "holding him back for a year" from school. It was their judgment that a year of extra help, and extra time for him to mature emotionally, would be beneficial to his progress in school. While it was true that he would no longer be in the same class as the children he'd known in kindergarten, and would in fact spend an extra year in the public school system, the upside could be much more considerable.

My wife and I considered the proposition, and eventually agreed with it. So Josh spent a year in Transitional Primary, which was probably his favorite year in school to date (at this writing, he is a freshman in high school, and doing quite well). He had time to mature a little, to understand the rules in school a little better and, because there was a teacher and a paraprofes-

Guns A'Blazing Discussion Questions

1. Note how often Cohen emphasizes the need for parents to advocate for their children to receive an education that is *equivalent*, not *better*, to the educational opportunities afforded their neuro-typical peers. How do you interpret "equal" versus "better" regarding educational programming for students with an autism spectrum disorder? Do you think that this is realistic advice to give to parents? Why does the author repeat this advice throughout the book?

2. What suggestions in the book did you disagree with, from the perspective of a teacher, a parent, or both? What would your recommendations be instead?

3. On page 125, Cohen writes: "An IEP meeting doesn't have to be something a parent dreads. With the right attitude and a little persistence, it's possible to enjoy the experience. Not incredibly likely, but possible." Reflect on your experiences as a participant in an IEP meeting, either as a parent or a teacher. Do you think that the majority of parents share this sentiment regarding IEP meetings, or is Cohen's opinion an exception to the rule? If parents are apprehensive about attending IEP meetings, what can we, as educators, do to make these experiences more positive?

4. Reflect on a situation involving conflict during a parent/teacher meeting that resulted in an unfavorable outcome. What information from this book would have been [illegible]

Release of Liability (2)

5. On pages 130-135 of the text, Cohen provides Tips for Teaching Higher Functioning People with Autism (reprinted by permission from Susan Moreno and Carol O' Neal.) Discuss how you could use this information to assist a colleague who is struggling to accommodate the needs of a student with autism.

6. As an educator, how can you use the information from this book to assist parents as they advocate for their children with special needs?
   As a parent, how will this information help you to better advocate for your child with special needs?

7. How has the information from Guns A'Blazing impacted your current practices and interactions with parents? How will this information guide your future practices when you participate in IEP meetings, either as a parent or educator?

sional in the room, he received more attention than he would have in the first-grade class he would have attended. Some of his classmates from kindergarten were in the class with him, and he established one friendship in that class that continues to the present day.

A long story, but what relevance does it have for you?

If my wife and I had stuck with our initial instincts, and opposed the suggestion based on our preconception that we were being treated with condescension, if we had kept our minds closed and not considered what was being offered, we would have done our son a great disservice. We could have let our own egos get in the way of what was best for him, gone in with Guns A' Blazing, and come out with precisely the opposite of what we really wanted – what was best for Josh.

I'm not telling you this story to give myself a pat on the back, especially since it was my wife who mostly talked me down off the ledge. The lesson to learn here is that it's possible to have too many expectations when you enter the school system, either public or private. Those who go through early intervention (which was not much of an option in 1995) are sometimes in for a rude awakening when they make the transition to a full-day program. The key is to do your homework ahead of time and understand what to expect when you walk in the first time to talk to a teacher, social worker, psychologist or administrator in the school system your child will attend.

Then, try to leave your expectations at the door, and listen.

It's entirely possible that you'll hear things you don't want to hear. In a coming chapter, we'll talk about the horror stories some parents have to tell. There are some school systems out there, both public and private, that do not understand how to handle children on the autism spectrum, and make outrageous suggestions or refuse to believe a child is eligible for the services he or she might require. I'm not saying that every school system is perfect and that you should do whatever they suggest. I am saying that the Guns A' Blazing approach is the wrong one to take on first contact. If you assume that the school system is the enemy, you've gone a long way toward making that the truth. It's possible that sort of relationship will develop over time, but there should be some benefit of the doubt initially on both parts. If you assume that you're in an adversarial relationship from the beginning, it's quite likely you will be correct. Conversely, if you assume that the professionals there are interested in doing what's right for every child in the system, it's possible that will turn out to be true as well.

Ellyn Atherton, who was the speech and language specialist in our school system when Josh was in kindergarten, and later became our district's director of educational services, is now director of human resources for the Springfield, New Jersey, school system. She says she understands, after hundreds of IEP meetings, why parents sometimes come into the system with negative expectations, but she recommends patience.

In fact, Atherton says that it's wise to get to know the members of the Child Study Team (or whatever group is to be involved in evaluating your child) before the first meeting. "Find someone who really understands your child, who spends time with him and 'gets' him, and you have found yourself an advocate," she advises.

In our case, Ellyn herself "got" Josh better than anyone else in the school system. She delighted in his humor and his unusual approach to life, and was always the person we sought out when there was a bump in the road. Even now, when she is no longer in the same school district, she will check in on Josh periodically, asking me about his progress.

One Pennsylvania mom agrees, telling me she finds that getting to know the people who will work with her 9-year-old son makes a tremendous difference. When her initial request for an IEP meeting was met with some resistance, she made it a point to talk to the school principal – but not about her son.

"I find out what makes that person tick by interviewing them," she explains. "I discovered (the principal) is an equestrian. So I found out where she keeps her horses, and I went out one afternoon and took pictures of her horses. I gave them to her, and (the principal) became my friend." The IEP meeting was scheduled.

Atherton says it's not simply a question of indulging every person's desire to be treated nicely. "In any relationship between people, there's going to be some resistance when the other person sees you're adversarial from the beginning," she says. "People always want to feel like they're being listened to, and that will lead to more people listening when you talk, as well."

The "Guns A' Blazing" approach is a natural reaction to the horror stories we hear when we first enter the autism community. It's hard, sometimes, to avoid the conclusion that teachers, principals, school psychologists and other school personnel are anything but welcoming when we arrive. And that can be a negative result of an otherwise very positive thing – the connection between parents of children on the spectrum.

When a child is diagnosed with autism, Asperger Syndrome or any related neurological condition, parents are quite often devastated. Some go into denial. Others immerse themselves in the information available, and often go to support group meetings or enter into Internet bulletin boards, mail lists and chat rooms. And that support, those connections, can go a long way toward making parents understand that they will survive this, and that their children can, very possibly, still achieve everything they hope for them.

But they also hear the horror stories. About school systems that won't cooperate, that are openly hostile to spectrum children and their families, that use restraints, lock children in closets or refuse to even discuss therapies or IEP meetings.

In such instances, sometimes the logical decision is to home school. That works well for a good number of people, and we will discuss it in much greater detail in a later chapter.

But for other parents, the horror stories are just that – horror stories. They are frightened and immediately assume that everything they hear from other parents – all of which is true – will also be the case for them. They make the logical jump from being told about bad situations (and very few good ones) to knowing that will be their experience. As a result, they dig in their heels and get ready for the long, tough battle they are sure is about to begin.

The problem is, they gear up for it before it happens, armed only with the information they have gathered through other people's experiences. They go in with Guns A' Blazing, assuming the "other side" is already as primed for battle as they are.

Sometimes they're right. But quite often, they're not.

To be fair, school districts do develop reputations within the autism/AS community. Knowing someone in your district (or private school) who has had experience can be helpful. It can tell you whom to approach ahead of time, and whom to avoid, in most cases. But there is no substitute for your own, personal experience, because you don't know how reasonable another parent might be in negotiations, and you don't know what everyone's circumstances are just through hearing them tell their story.

Be prepared, and do your homework. Know the people you'll be dealing with. Have a reasonable list of services your child truly needs (we'll discuss that at length later), and go in knowing that you might have to hold back a little at first and listen more than you talk.

If your experience ends up like my son's, the preparation will be well worth it. If it doesn't, there are alternatives, as we will discuss.

Keep that weapon in your holster, soldier. The battle has not yet begun.

Chapter Two

HORROR STORIES

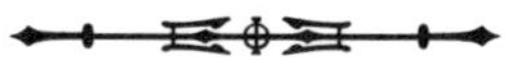

"We started having problems with him being given suspensions and detentions, and they would stick him in a room near the teachers' lounge and leave him there for hours on end unsupervised." One Nebraska woman remembers the problems her 9-year-old son, then with a preliminary diagnosis of Asperger Syndrome, had in fourth grade. The district, which was enforcing a zero-tolerance policy on behavior, failed to understand that frustration and anger may be signs of a neurological disorder, and not simply a behavioral problem.

"The school district was aware we were looking for a diagnosis, and finally there was a day when just nothing was going right, and (my son) was having meltdown after meltdown after meltdown, and finally used some threatening language. The principal, at that point, said 'he's making terroristic threats,' so she called his grandmother to come pick him up."

The boy sat in the car silently for a long time that October afternoon, until he finally turned to his grandmother and said, "I think I'll just go out as myself this Halloween, because I'm scary."

We all hear the horror stories, and we all have them: either tiny, insignificant ones, or more serious incidents that can threaten a child's education, his relationship with the school system, and sometimes even his psychological state. The Nebraska mom's son was clinically depressed at age 9, she says four years later, but his parents and the school system were unaware of it at the time.

"They said he had to have a one-on-one aide because he was a violent child and a ticking time bomb," she remembers. "We were in an absolute panic. I did not feel he was safe in (the school) building. We home schooled him for three months."

The boy's parents eventually opted to send him to another public school district in the area, where he is receiving services and thriving at this writing.

No school system, from home schooling to the New York City public school system, is perfect, but some are more imperfect than others. Sometimes parents expect too much from a school district. Those aren't the cases we're discussing in this chapter.

These are horror stories. I'm not going to tell you all the ones I've heard from parents with children on the autism spectrum, not only because it would take up the whole book, but also because there's a danger of expecting this kind of behavior, even from a school district that is truly trying to do what's best for the child with autism or Asperger Syndrome. But a few stories, illustrating the kind of difficulties parents have faced with teachers and administrators who don't understand the spectrum, might help us understand why the relationship between some parents and some schools is, let's say, less than ideal.

There have been children held in restraints in schoolrooms and on school buses. There has been a child suspended from school for kicking a teacher in the shin, even when the child had no history of physical aggression and insisted he did no such thing, with no witness present. After the 9/11 attacks, some schools with "zero-tolerance" policies have been less willing to understand the disorder that causes a child to lose control when he is frustrated, or to use language that the school might consider a "terroristic threat," with no intention of doing any such thing.

But there are other horror stories, too. These are the ones that go on between parents and school districts in a struggle to get proper services for a child on the autism spectrum. Speech and language therapy, occupational therapy, social skills training and other services are sometimes the source of bitter contention between schools and parents, and those stories, while less graphic, are just as disturbing, because they indicate a problem that the educational system has with children who don't fit the mold, especially when it comes to being "socially acceptable."

My son has never been suspended from school, but that's a minor miracle. In his time, which thankfully was several years ago, he managed to avoid suspension while still threatening a teacher, choking a classmate and, in a masterstroke only a week after the 9/11 attacks occurred less than an hour's drive from our home, letting slip that he wouldn't mind burning the school down. (Skip ahead to Chapter Sixteen for more on that one.)

Luckily, our school district understood the disorder with which my son contends every day. Our son's IEP includes a clause insisting that we be consulted before any authorities are called if he disrupts the class in an inappropriate manner, which luckily hasn't happened in a few years. Other school districts have been known to call the police, in a show of zero tolerance, even when they know the child in question is not intending to do harm to himself or anyone else. But from the school's point of view, it's understandable that a child who can't control himself with a classmate, or verbally threatens a staff member, could be "the one" who slips through the cracks, and the principal or teacher who looks the other way because "he's such a nice boy most of the time" might be ignoring a very serious problem. It's a tough line to walk.

In our case, the problem never became very serious. But when a situation is developing, there is no way to know how it will play out, and that leads to behavior by school personnel that sometimes seems far more alarmist than the event itself merits.

"(My son)'s reactions are not appropriate," one Oregon woman told me. "He'd be throwing Legos, or hitting somebody.

We told (the principal) about our concerns. Things just went downhill. That school (private school) so much wanted to please parents that they wouldn't tell you when something happened. I'm thinking everything's going fine. We were very honest; we didn't leave anything out.

"When things got worse, and (the boy) became 'out of control' (in the school's terminology), he had what I would call a complete meltdown, and wound up breaking his hand by pounding his fist into the ground over and over," his mother recalls. "The principal took away his coat hook in the room. We thought that doesn't make him feel like he's part of the class."

Advised by the child's doctor, his parents moved him to the public school system in their area and requested appropriate services. "He started out doing okay in that honeymoon period, but as soon as that thought creeps into my head, it starts going downhill," his mother says. "He's been suspended five times in three months. The principal does not want my child in that school. I found out that one of the school staff pinched him. To me, that sounds like a restraint, like you're trying to calm somebody down. No restraints are approved in his IEP. Somebody had to make a split-second decision, and I'm not questioning that, but I should have been informed, and it didn't cross their minds to call me."

How could this pattern have been avoided? The key to almost every successful interaction between parents and schools is communication. The fact that "it didn't cross their minds to call" is key here. That's what sticks in the mother's mind, and that's what she doesn't understand.

Sometimes, school personnel feel it's best to show that they are more than capable of handling every situation, that they don't need to bother busy parents in the course of a day. But parents of children on the spectrum need to, by definition, be more involved in the day-to-day dealings of their children than parents of most neurotypical kids. We want to be told when a situation has arisen, because we might be able to help defuse it faster and more successfully than others. Especially when our children are younger, we spend much more time with them than anyone else, and we know their moods and their behaviors. We can help, and we're happy to do so.

We're thrilled when we get a report from the school that everything's going well. But when everything isn't going well, we need to know quickly.

As a parent, you can't rely on teachers or school personnel to know that you're available when needed. You have to insist that they contact you. My son's IEP includes a sentence that promotes and encourages communication with the home (which is me, generally, since I work in the house). We make sure each of his teachers knows it's there, and I hand out business cards at the beginning of the year with my phone number, my cell phone number, my wife's office number and all our email addresses, above and beyond the information forms the school distributes to parents at the beginning of every academic year.

Periodically, I email his teachers, asking if there are any concerns they want to discuss. I do this because you never know if something is going on unless you ask – many teachers are reluctant to tell a parent, thinking they can handle the situation, or that the parent doesn't want to be bothered.

This strategy is almost always a recipe for disaster. School systems that act as a team with parents succeed, and those that act as independent, sometimes competing, entities from parents very rarely succeed. Simple.

A key for parents is to anticipate and have provisions included in the IEP. This is never simple, since it's impossible to anticipate many situations that might arise with a child on the spectrum. Even parents with some experience dealing with schools forget certain possibilities or don't see the signs before their children exhibit a new behavior or react to a situation that hasn't come up before.

"(My daughter) comes home every day without the right books, without the right homework," says a mother from Toronto, Canada. "It's a daily struggle. I know what she needs and what to do. We were sitting in a meeting one day and the vice principal suddenly said, 'I know! Why don't we give her two sets of textbooks!' That's been in every document I've ever written for the past five years."

For Asperger Syndrome children and those with high-functioning autism, organization can be a huge struggle. School systems that don't "get it" can place their emphasis on the wrong area, assuming the problem is a behavioral one.

"I could tell something was wrong," says one North Dakota mom. "It's hard for him to raise his hand and say, 'I need help.' I wanted to call an IEP meeting, but they didn't know if we should do that. They got together, and the principal came up with the idea that we should use cards. (My son's) aide put some words on his cards that he can keep in his desk. One was 'I need a break,' another, 'I don't understand,' and yet another, 'I need help.' He just puts that on his desk.

"Last year, the teacher said he was doing so well and we should see what he can do, and (my son) ended up with an ulcer," she continues. "He felt like he couldn't go down to the aide for help because he was under pressure to perform in the classroom."

Some school systems appear resistant to any accommodations made for students on the autism spectrum. Without a formal diagnosis, it's difficult to get any services, and sometimes that means hiring a consultant, an advocate or an attorney to come in to argue the child's case from the parents' point of view.

Each state and country has its own laws concerning the process, but the undeniable truth is that when a dispute between a parent and a school system reaches the court system, the situation isn't good.

Indeed, often by then, the situation has degenerated from being about a child's education and is often about the personal animosity between the parents and the school officials. At that point, the objective, emotionless view of an outside consultant may be just the thing the situation needs.

For a parent, an objective perspective is difficult to maintain. Raising a child isn't a series of intellectual decisions; it generally comes from a more emotional place, and stirs great passions. Anyone who tells the parent of a child with autism or Asperger Syndrome "no" had best expect a reaction that doesn't necessarily stem from the highest-functioning part of the brain.

Does that make parents wrong when they question a school system? Of course not. It means that any interaction between humans is likely to stir some sort of emotion, and when one or more of those humans are parents of a child on the spectrum, the emotions are likely to be more intense, motivated by a desire to protect that child.

The horror stories are helpful because they teach us what can go wrong, and point out ways to avoid that – those who came before us are marking the way and showing us where the danger lies. But the horror stories are not a foregone conclusion; they don't have to be expected as much as anticipated. Parents who go in with Guns A' Blazing aren't likely to avoid the horror stories. Indeed, they are more likely to become part of the next one.

Don't try to become a cautionary tale. Work hard and push for what your child needs, but let the system fail you before you condemn it as a failure.

Chapter Three

INCLUSION VS. ISOLATION

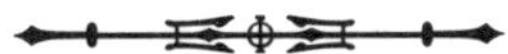

Few decisions the parent of a child with special needs has to make are more basic than where the child will attend school. Rarely a simple choice, it is often one that impacts on the child's education from the beginning to adulthood.

For parents who have decided on a public school system, or who can't afford any alternative (if local school systems are unwilling or unable to pay for a private placement), another question immediately follows: should the child with autism or Asperger Syndrome be included in a class with neurotypical children (a "mainstream" class), or should the child be in a separate, special education classroom, where he or she will be learning with other children who have reasons not to be in the mainstream class?

This is not the last time you'll hear this from me: I'm not going to tell you what choice to make, because I don't know your child. But I will detail for you what each choice means, and perhaps illustrate it with examples of people who have made each choice (and in some cases, have made both choices at one time or another). While parents may not be able to make the ultimate decision, they can choose what they want to request, and their request can become more insistent as IEPs are written and hearings are held, if necessary.

My son has been in a public school system from the time he first entered what was then called "Pre-K Handicapped" to the present day, when he is a high school student. We never considered asking for him to be in a special needs class, and the school never suggested it.

However, when he was slated for the transitional primary class I mentioned in Chapter One, we had the quick moment of disagreement I wrote about. There was considerable talk at the time about a child being "stigmatized" because of a diagnosis, a classification in the public school system or a "label," such as "autistic" or "special needs." It was a scary possibility, and one that took a good deal of convincing to sell.

Thank goodness the school personnel were able to explain it properly, because the transitional year was the most valuable tool my son has ever had. It fit him perfectly, and gave him exactly what he needed at that age to be able to handle most of what was to come in the following school years (not all, by any stretch of the imagination, but most).

Still, the very suggestion that Josh should have to spend a year outside the "mainstream," that he should be isolated from the classmates he'd met and spent a rather difficult kindergarten year getting to know, was troubling. He was 6 years old, and already had enough difficulty making friends. Taking him away from the only children he'd known in school so far seemed to be something other than the best possible course of action for him.

Now take that, and imagine it as a full-time decision without a distinct limit in terms of time. Imagine that the school is suggesting your child be isolated from the rest of the school community for the foreseeable future, and unless significant social skills (or other) progress is made, maintain that placement for his or her entire school career.

There are two schools (pardon the expression) of thought on the subject. One, the knee-jerk reaction that the child will be lonely, will not be able to progress socially by constant exposure to other children who aren't progressing socially, and will therefore be alienated, "branded" and teased throughout school, is natural.

But so is the thought that a lot of parents with children on the spectrum have: one of distinct relief. Thank goodness your child won't have to compete socially with neurotypical classmates. Thank goodness your child will be able to find friends among those more closely suited to his ability and emotional maturity level. Thank goodness the teasing might stop.

Either one of those reactions is understandable and defensible. Either one makes sense, and either one can be perfect for your child, as you know your child's abilities and personality best. But if you're not sure, if the thought of one alternative or the other doesn't immediately ring a bell in your head that says, "of course!," you run the risk of guilt and doubt – if you make the choice, and it turns out to be the wrong one ...

Well, then you can change your mind. It's not easy to get a school system to reverse course, but it's possible, and in most cases, legally mandated. Your child must, in most states and most countries, be in the school environment that suits him best.

If the school is reluctant to change the current situation, think about the reason. Yes, you know your child better than anyone else, but here's a secret few will tell you: Children at home are different than children at school. At the early school conferences in October, I hear my daughter's teachers tell me about what a quiet, reserved, shy child she is and I have to bite my tongue to keep from laughing. At home, we can barely get a word in edgewise. And by the end of the school year, they'll be talking about how gregarious, outgoing and talkative she is in class. Kids aren't the same wherever they go. So it's possible that your child's behavior in school is not the same as what you're used to at home.

It's also possible the school has good reasons to keep your child in the current program. Maybe her teachers are seeing progress academically that neither of you expected. Maybe behavioral issues haven't improved yet, but the school psychologist is seeing signs that they might soon. Maybe the expected improvement from moving the child to another program is impaired by the shock to his system: Children on the spectrum (I don't need to tell you) are not crazy about change. Will moving to another type of classroom, with all new classmates, a new teacher and a new style of teaching, be offset by enough improvement to merit the change? It's something you have to decide.

Still, change is possible; don't rule it out simply because the school says no. If you do all the evaluations and decide that your child isn't in the right program now, be it inclusive or special, you need to make the change.

But how do you make that decision?

The argument to be made in favor of inclusion classrooms is strong. Children on the spectrum might learn social skills through exposure to neurotypical classmates. They are quite often on, or above, grade level academically and should be allowed to flourish in their studies, something which may or may not be likely in a special needs class. (Again, generalization is a dangerous, inaccurate thing – I'm not saying that children who aren't in mainstream classes are definitely not going to have the same academic opportunities, just that it's something to investigate.)

On the other hand, there is a very strong case to be made for certain children on the spectrum being taught outside the mainstream class. Some, because of an accelerated academic ability, should be in classes for gifted children (the incidence of giftedness is significant in children on the spectrum). Some need help academically and can't keep up the pace that would be required in a mainstream classroom. Others still would be perfectly at home academically in a traditional class, but would have so much difficulty sitting still long enough, or dealing with peers in social situations, that keeping them in included classes could be counterproductive or damaging.

This is a classic situation in which the decision should be made by the parents, but the school personnel should be consulted, with a sympathetic ear. It's not always easy to hear what someone is telling you about your child (think of when you heard the word "autism" in relation to your child for the first time), but that doesn't mean anything you haven't considered yourself should be dismissed out of hand. Communication between the school and you, the parents, is essential in all dealings when a child on the spectrum is involved. This is a central decision, and you can't make it all on your own. You need the information that only those who spend their time dealing with children in school – and your child in school, all day – can have.

The hardest part of communication is listening. It's easy to tell others what you think is the right way to go – it's not that easy to hear an opinion that might conflict with you own. When both parties in the conversation are willing to consider both viewpoints, something can be done. The truth generally lies in the middle, after all.

If the school's principal, or the team working with you, disagrees with your conclusion, that's not necessarily a sign of conflict; it may be a difference of opinion, or it may be that one side or the other hasn't gotten all the information it needs yet – and that includes you.

Keep both ears open, and make sure the teachers, administrators and Child Study Team do the same. One of my favorite quotes is from the actor/writer/director Alan Alda, who said his philosophy of life is: "Be fair with others, but then keep after them until they're fair with you."

That means not looking for ways to be insulted, not seeing "hidden meanings" in everything that's said, and not backing down just because someone tells you "that isn't the way it's done." What they really mean (and they might not know it) is: "That isn't the way it's been done ... yet."

Be well prepared with an opinion about which type of class would be best for your child. Do the research, and consider your child's personality. Then walk into the meeting with the school's representatives, and listen. Don't assume the matter has been settled ahead of time; if my wife and I had done that with our son's second year in school, as mentioned, he'd have missed out on a valuable tool that has served him well in the nine years since then. But present your reasoning – your opinion and how you arrived at it – and listen to the responses. If the people you're talking to clearly aren't hearing what you're saying, restate it politely. Getting angry won't help anyone, least of all your child.

One parent from West Virginia told me her son had "bounced back and forth between the mainstream class and the special ed class three times" before finally staying in a mainstream classroom. The difference was changing teachers. "(He) really hated the first teacher, and I got the feeling she didn't like him," she says. "But in the special ed room, his behavior was modeling on the other kids in the class, and he was talking less at home. When we moved him to the new mainstream class, he and the teacher just clicked, and that made the difference. He's doing great now."

Unfortunately, it took two separate changes in the child's life to find him the right place to be, and his mother continues to worry: "What's going to happen next year? I'm going to have to get to know the teachers in advance this time."

We make mistakes, and we learn from them. That's a lesson we can teach our children that will help them through their lives.

Preparation, as in all things on the spectrum, is essential. Get to know the teachers involved. Talk to other parents, particularly those whose children have special needs. Find out which teachers are more willing to deal with differences, and lobby hard until you can be sure your child will be in their class. And constantly monitor the situation.

"It never stops," the West Virginia mom says. "You can't ever just relax."

But if you know you made your decision thoughtfully and objectively, maybe you can sleep better at night.

Of course, sometimes, it's possible to have it both ways. The New York City school system has begun running two schools (one in Brooklyn, the other on Staten Island) that cater specifically to the growing population of high-functioning children with autism spectrum disorders, in particular Asperger Syndrome. Steve Rosen, director of Special Education for District 8 (which houses both schools) says parents drove the push for the schools, and the city responded.

"Children with high-functioning autism were not doing as well as we thought they should," he reports. "We spent a year studying this, and with the help of some of the parents and the program at the Jewish Community Center in Fort Lee (New Jersey), we decided we can do a better job."

The schools combine classes that include only children with autism spectrum disorders with times during the day when those students are integrated into the mainstream population of the school.

"There are two different types of classes," Rosen says. "There are NEST classes, in which we do a lot of social stories and other social skills tools, and then there are the usual academic classes, and sometimes, the children in the NEST classes work with children in the included classes."

In some classes, there are eight typically developing children, eight with high-functioning autism and two teachers, Rosen says. "We have to change to meet the needs of the kids," he says. "We've seen children turn around within a year." The program is expected to reach the fifth-grade level, "and if we have to take it to middle school, we will," Rosen adds.

If a school system as large and complex as that in New York City can make major accommodations, there is hope for all of us. Decide what's right for your child, and then push until someone listens.

Chapter Four

PUBLIC VS. PRIVATE

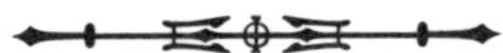

Most people on a middle-class income rely on the public school systems in their communities to educate their children. They provide an education that, depending on the community and the school system, gives the area's children at the very least the mandated education specified by local, state and federal guidelines. It works just fine for most people.

But most people don't have a child on the autism spectrum.

Children with social skills, educational and overall life issues stemming from a neurological condition have needs related to school that are not the same as those of neurotypical peers. That's basic. That's logical. But it's not always obvious.

When the child has Asperger Syndrome, for example, his needs might not be immediately noticeable. My son can function quite "normally" in a school environment, as long as the situation remains predictable and structured. If something out of the ordinary occurs, however, his behavior will not necessarily fall in line with that of his classmates. But it might. There's no way to predict it in advance.

That's why he has special accommodations from the school system.

As of this writing, Josh has a full-time, one-on-one aide named Joyce Gregus, who stays with him through his school day. Mrs. Gregus doesn't often have to intercede on Josh's behalf, as they've been together in school for seven years. But she knows the warning signs, she knows the situations that are especially likely to upset him, and she knows what to do when those situations present themselves. Mrs. Gregus is my son's safety net, and while she might not be needed now as much as when he was in third grade, when she is needed, she's needed.

Her presence is an accommodation from the public school system, which recognized early on that my son would require some help in order to get the same education – not a better one or a different one – as his neurotypical peers. The school psychologist, social worker, special education teacher and speech and language therapist who met Josh when he was in kindergarten no longer work for the town's school system, but their initial work put in place the supports that still exist for him, and will for as long as they are needed, until he graduates from the school system and (we hope) goes on to college. I often joke with Mrs. Gregus that she'll have to room with him at college, and there are days I think she'd go along with that plan. Well, she'd stay in the same dormitory, anyway.

There are distinct advantages to availing yourself of the public school system in your community. Chief among these is that the public school system is, aside from the taxes that support it (and which you have to pay whether your child goes to the public school or not), free. This is not a flippant comment, nor is it meant to insinuate that public schools deliver a lesser education or fewer services, but to suggest that economic issues make them attractive to those who can't afford an alternative. But, consider that to send a child to a school for students with special needs in my town can cost upwards of $30,000 per year for tuition and transportation, and the public school my son attends costs me ... nothing, and you see the issue.

Beyond that, public schools in many areas are indeed more fully equipped to deal with the needs of a student on the autism spectrum than some private schools (home schooling is another matter, which we'll discuss in a later chapter). They have done so more often than many private schools, are required to make accommodations by law, and have support staff regulated and mandated by law who are required to educate every child in the system.

Of course, that is a best-case scenario. As the parents with Horror Stories can tell you, just because something is supposed to be handled in a certain way, you shouldn't necessarily expect it to be handled that way. Rather, school administrators, even teachers, sometimes interpret the rules their own way, and some are not as knowledgeable about the education of children with autism spectrum disorders as they would be in a world we would create. Indeed, as more diagnoses are made, some teachers and school officials seem to see spectrum parents as a special-interest group with unreasonable demands that simply doesn't seem to understand how to discipline a child.

Public schools, like any other public institution, are not perfect. They are maddeningly variable. Thus, parents often find that moving a child from one district to another, from one school to another within the district, and even from one class to another within the same school, can mean enormous changes, based on the personalities of teachers and children, and often, those of parents and administrators. Going in with Guns A' Blazing can make enemies, and once the first pistol is drawn, it's awfully hard to get them all safely back into holsters without a shot being fired.

Private schools fall under two extremely general categories: "mainstream" private schools that are not specialized in their focus for children on the spectrum, and "special needs" schools that make an effort to concentrate specifically on children with autism, AS or related conditions.

Some mainstream private schools are parochial schools or preparatory schools. While they have probably had some experience with the autism spectrum, it is not their main focus. Some might be equipped to deal with a child who has autism issues, others might not.

And here is a cold, cruel truth about all private schools: They can accept the children they are willing to include, and decline to accept others. There is no governmental hierarchy requiring them to accept every child who applies. It's like college – if they want you, you can attend.

If the school is willing to consider a child on the spectrum, it's imperative that the parents make very clear to a private school (or a public school, for that matter) what can be expected from their child. If he has specific sensitivities to loud noises, certain smells (which can be a challenge around lunch time) or other sensory distractions, don't let the school personnel find out about it for themselves – tell them in advance. If the child has a history of aggressive behavior (my son was a biter in his early school years, ever in his quest for the least socially acceptable way to act out), don't conceal the information: The school will find out on its own, and if there is honesty at the beginning, teachers and staff can be on the lookout for sensitive situations, and perhaps prevent a few incidents.

Private schools that concentrate on children with special needs or those that work exclusively with children on the spectrum are less likely to be surprised by any behavior the child will exhibit. When deciding on a school, the question is the same as that posed in the previous chapter: Do you want your child in an environment with peers who are neurotypical, or with those who also are on the autism spectrum?

It's unfortunate, but often the choice is an economic one. "My husband is known as the 'Candy Man' at our IEP meetings," one public school mom told me. "We're not paying for private school, so we can afford a lot of candy." Private schools in general are not inexpensive, and those with a special interest in the spectrum can be even more expensive. Still, there are alternatives.

Some of the most heated arguments between parents and school systems come when the parents request an out-of-district placement, or for the school system to pay private school tuition (and in many cases, transportation) for a child. These can become contentious battles, particularly when a school system is not inclined to agree that the child won't do well enough in public school, and the parents believe otherwise.

I know of one child in New Jersey whose parents were asked to allow him to attend a private school in another town. The school district, which claimed to be unable to handle the boy, was willing to pay a large tuition every year as well as the cost for the transportation (an hour in each direction) that would be necessary for the child to attend the school, one specializing in autism spectrum conditions.

The parents, at first, were hesitant: What was this school system trying to pull on them? But after a good deal of conversation, they let their son give the private school a try – and he's still there, four years later.

"I was skeptical, but he loves it, and he's doing really well," his mother told me. "Sometimes, we're a little paranoid that if the idea comes from the school, it can't be good for our children. But this one was."

Most of the time, the situation is the reverse – parents trying to persuade a school system, whose budget is strained to begin with, to pay tuition at a private school. It can be hard to make the case. Public schools are not crazy about paying a lot of money for a child to be placed elsewhere. But when they agree that the child will not do well in public school (or when enough problems with behavior have made the point obvious), agreements can be reached.

Another mother here in New Jersey told me that she and her school system could not reach an agreement on her daughter's placement, so she ended up finding a middle ground between public and private schools. "She's in a co-op school now," she says. "We moved her there in the second grade (two years ago).

She's keeping up in class work now. You pay less tuition than some private schools, but you have a parent job, and you're involved. But it's still (a good deal of money). Wouldn't you know it, my daughter wants to go back to public school now."

There's no easy way to persuade a school system to send your child outside the district. Sometimes parents have found that requesting a change in schools within the district can make enough of a difference. In some states, it's possible to request a transfer to another school, and sometimes the rules allow for one change within the state with no questions asked. However, even when an open enrollment situation is available, it's not always easy to know which school to request.

As with most things in being a parent with a child on the spectrum, it's important to communicate with other parents. Get to know the other parents in your district (and other nearby districts) whose children are diagnosed with conditions similar to your child's. Find out what they like and what they don't like about their schools. Discover who the "open-minded" teachers are, and request them by name. If you need to make a request for a placement outside the current school or in another district, know which options are best for your child. But have backup plans ready if what you are requesting isn't available.

For those who can afford it, and whose public school systems are unwilling to pay for it, private school is a helpful alternative. Some parents whose children fit into the "gifted" category prefer to have them taught at schools that are especially equipped to educate children with unusual or notable talents in academic fields. Often, with children who have Asperger Syndrome, their "special interest" can be indulged a bit more in private schools, possibly becoming a source of pride and strength for the child.

Other parents are committed to the idea of a public school education, and sometimes have to fight a little harder for the services their children require, but don't have to pay private school tuitions or worry that their children will not be allowed to attend school at all. Still others opt for a completely separate alternative.

For them, school and home are the same thing.

Chapter Five

HOW ABOUT NO SCHOOL AT ALL?

Sometimes the strain of trying to deal with a school – any school – can be overwhelming for an autism spectrum parent. Teachers don't (or don't want to) understand why a perfectly "normal-looking" child with "behavior problems" needs special accommodations; principals worry about the budgetary consequences of providing a full-time aide, social skills services and, in some cases, at-home therapies or out-of-district placement for one child when hundreds of others need attention, too. In some cases, even social workers, psychologists and therapists seem to be in opposition to the needs of a child on the spectrum.

The bureaucracy can be daunting, at best, and the rules of appeal – from teacher to principal to superintendent to school board, through mediation to due process hearing – can be labyrinthine and time-consuming. Sometimes, it seems like there is no alternative but caving in and letting the school do what it pleases.

But, there is.

For some parents, home schooling is the best thing they've ever considered. Their children are well taught by people who understand their autism and Asperger Syndrome, and who love them to boot. Many families believe the practice has made them closer, and improved the children's education.

Home schooling is an experience that combines all the usual aspects of parenting a child on the autism spectrum with the additional responsibilities of teacher, principal and school superintendent. For some parents, it is an exhilarating, enriching and rewarding experience that they couldn't imagine giving up.

For others, it is an alternative that, frankly, is too much responsibility, or simply out of the question financially (at least one parent has to be home every day and, generally speaking, that means a one-income family).

Again, I'm not here to decide for you. I've never attempted home schooling, so I can't tell you what my opinion is, since I have none. I can tell you about the parents I've interviewed, and how they view their experiences. And those run in both directions.

"I tried it and it was a disaster," one parent from Israel told me. "(My son) needed a real, regulated framework. I tried, my husband tried, it cost us thousands of dollars (in lost income), and it just didn't work."

On the other hand, a mother from Pennsylvania said she has "always felt home schooling is intriguing. I really like it. There are days when, like every other parent, you want to pull your hair out. But I enjoy education; that's my field, and a lot of school districts are not supportive. The bigger ones don't even care (about spectrum children)."

As these perspectives suggest, home schooling is the kind of thing that some parents seem to adore and others recoil from. Those who like it love it, and those who don't probably have never seriously considered doing it. Few are lukewarm in their opinion on the subject, however. There's little middle ground.

The bottom line is if you can afford to home school, and think it's something you would enjoy doing, it's another alternative. If you get dizzy at the very suggestion of it, no matter how much grief you're getting from your school district, the odds are you're not going to enjoy it, and that means you'll probably not do it well, and consequently you won't be doing your child any favors.

The arguments in favor of home schooling are persuasive: Your child gets exactly the education you think she should have. She gets it from someone who is devoted exclusively to her needs and, therefore, can tailor the curriculum to her strengths and weaknesses. There are no classmates (unless you're home schooling siblings as well), so there will be no teasing (see previous parenthetical expression). The stress level (for your child) is low, as she will be in familiar surroundings, will understand every aspect of the routine, and won't have to go to the lunchroom at noon with hundreds of schoolmates – unless you have an extremely large kitchen.

"I had decided we were going to do it (home school) for a while because (my son) doesn't deal well with large groups," says the Pennsylvania-based home schooling mom. "He does much better in a small group." Her son's two siblings are also being home schooled, although they are at different grade levels.

Parents who home school don't merely wake up one morning and decide it's time for algebra. Very specific, extremely detailed curricula are available for review from most libraries and a growing number of home schooling organizations. In many cases, some funding for books is available from the local or state school board. There are organizations of home schoolers, many on the Internet and many specializing in autism spectrum home schooling. (Since I have no firsthand knowledge of the groups, I'm not recommending any of them, but if you run a Google search with the keywords "home school," "autism" and "organization," you should get a very large representative group.)

For children on the autism spectrum, particularly those with high-functioning autism or Asperger Syndrome, social interaction with peers is often a serious issue at school, and home schooling is a way to reduce that stress. But some parents argue that removing the child from the school environment doesn't so much solve the problem of socialization as it postpones it, and gives the child even less time to develop the necessary skills as he grows.

"Socialization is too big a part of what (my son) needs to master," says one parent in Texas. "Plus, if he needs to survive in the 'real world'/a real work place, he has to learn to get along and to interact with his neurotypical peers. He would not get that if he were home schooled."

Not surprisingly, there is no consensus on the question of socialization for children being home schooled. Parents who are home schooling their children point to local groups of home-schooled children who get together on a regular basis for field trips or social outings, and say that interaction with other children sharing the same experience helps their own children get the peer interaction they need.

"I'm a certified educator, and I do evaluations for other home schoolers," says the Pennsylvania mom. "We've gotten to know other home schooling families, and we get together sometimes."

In some cases, the outings are more organized than they would be in a public school, and socialization is a specific curriculum item. But parents who home school are often puzzled by the emphasis many place on what has been a source of great stress for their children.

"They're going to learn about the world by being in the world," one Michigan home schooling parent told me. "(My son) spent years in public school being teased and bullied by other kids, and that was the terrific experience he was supposed to be having? At home, he doesn't have the stress, and he doesn't come home crying every day."

Tammy Glaser is a Colorado mom who decided to home school her daughter in 1995 after three years in preschool special education in the local school system. "I was frustrated because, out of those three years, she had only one year in which things clicked for her," she recalls. "I realized that I would never be 'guaranteed' an ideal teacher and would waste valuable time every time (my daughter) transitioned to a new teacher. And the noise and chaos of a typical classroom and school hindered her ability to function."

Glaser began schooling her daughter at home, and after 10 years now advises other home schoolers through her website http://home.earthlink.net/~tammyglaser798/authome.html. She founded Aut 2B Home, an email list dedicated to the home schooling of children on the spectrum.

Still, Glaser understands that not all children or all parents are perfect for home schooling. She doesn't get involved in arguments about the subject, preferring instead to advise those who ask. "As with anything in the autism world ... one can waste energy arguing heatedly over what is 'best' or one can get on with doing what is best for your unique child," she told me. "The way I see it, parents are smart enough to discern what educational options work best for their children. What works best for my kids and my personal situation may not work best for their kids and their personal situation. As long as my decisions are treated with respect, I am fully prepared to respect the decisions of home schooling and non-home schooling parents. Whether their kids are in school or are schooled at home, I support the fact that the parents have taken the time to make a choice, and do what they think is best for their kids."

Glaser says, however, that she does not believe children schooled at home are missing out on socialization opportunities, and offers her own daughter as an example: "We go to the library (three times a week. My daughter) has to interact with the librarians to ask for a computer and check out books. She has to be respectful of any adults she meets ... we walk everywhere, so she has to learn street smarts, crossing streets, riding the bus, and so on, while we are out. She also has many opportunities to interact with other children. She takes two co-op classes. One night a week, she goes to dinner at church (meeting every age group) and sings in the kids' choir. Once a week, she takes a home school recreation class ... her experiences are richer because she gets to interact with kids of a variety of ages. She gets the best of both worlds."

The idea that children should only interact with peers their own age is questionable, Glaser believes. "Actually, when you think about it, we adults do not socialize with peers primarily in our own age group," she says. "Since I graduated from college, I don't run around in packs of people about my age. In real life, I meet all kinds of people from all walks of life. What happens to some children in school is they learn to focus primarily on kids their own age, and they lose the ability to relate to adults, younger children, the elderly, and so forth. The beauty of home schooling is that children are able to socialize with people of a variety of ages, not just their peers."

Because parents are able to construct the class in any way they feel is best, home schoolers can be as conventional (or unconventional) as they please. Glaser says that the one-on-one attention parents can give to home-schooled children is a great benefit, particularly to children on the autism spectrum, but she doesn't advocate one type of home schooling over another; she believes individualization is a benefit, not a drawback.

"I generally recommend that interested parents read books written for beginner home schoolers. They are chock full of things to consider, such as reading state laws to enable parents to home school legally," she says. "Parents usually imagine setting up school at home (textbook/workbook on an exact schedule). While this approach works for some kids, other kids fail to thrive. So it's helpful to learn about the wide variety of philosophies on how to home school (unit studies, classical, literature-based, Waldorf, Montessori, un-schooling, etc.).

"Some parents find that figuring out the learning styles of everyone (parents and children) can help them target the most effective way of learning."

She recommends the books *So You're Thinking About Homeschooling* by Lisa Whelchel, *The Way They Learn and Every Child Can Succeed* by Cynthia Tobias and *Discover Your Child's Learning Style* by Mariaemma Willis and Victoria Kindle-Hodson, among others.

"There are also books and websites which provide guidelines of what information and skills need to be mastered by grade level," Glaser says. "Because every family finds their own way of doing things, what you might see happening in my home may be quite different from the other home schooling families who live in my town."

Home schooling is not a fad, and it's not a withdrawal from society; it's a choice. Even the most ardent proponents of the practice won't argue that it's the right choice for every child, or the right choice for every child on the autism spectrum. But it is a choice, and if it fits your child perfectly enough, it might be something you'd like to consider.

Chapter Six

WHAT TO ASK FOR

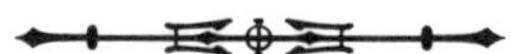

When parents are faced, for the first time, with the idea that their child might have a disorder on the autism spectrum, they are overwhelmed. Not many "laypeople" understand the wide spectrum of behaviors that autism can encompass, and our views of it as presented in popular culture are not, let's say, one hundred percent accurate. Think *Rainman.*

At that first moment, there is a lot of data to absorb. Just the fact that there's something your child will have to deal with all his life – something that most children never have to consider – is enough to cause a good deal of sleeplessness. Once you get past that idea (which in many cases can take some time), you have to consider exactly what has to be done in order to help level the playing field for your child.

There is some debate in the autism community as to what the best course of action is. Some believe that autism is not something that needs to be "cured" or "controlled," but that it is a personality type, and that the problem is society's. This is a valid point of view, but for the sake of our purposes here, I'm going to assume that you want your child to fit into the accepted version of society as much as possible, and work from that premise.

Your dealings with your school system will be colored by your child's specific needs. That is to say, there is no secret formula of services that will be right for every child on the spectrum, not even every child with the same diagnosis. Personality plays a role, and a significant one, in determining what each child needs to get the same education as everyone else in school.

Some will benefit from a full-time, one-on-one aide, as my son has. Others would find such an arrangement embarrassing and stifling, and would perform worse, rather than better, under those circumstances. Your child's personality will be a factor in determining what kind of help he might need.

This is a key point: You're not trying to get your child a better education than the other children attending her school. For one thing, no school system will agree to that. Public schools are not required to provide such a thing (assuming it even exists), and it would, under any circumstances, be unfair and indefinable. You are approaching the school with ideas for services that you think will make school possible for your child, to make it possible for her to receive an education equivalent to that offered her neurotypical peers. It's important to stress that, since any appearance that we're trying to get an unrealistic set of services from a school system will be met with a negative response from virtually every school on the planet, and won't gain us any allies among school personnel or other parents in our community.

That said, how do you determine what services are necessary? How can your child really get that level playing field and the same chance as everyone else in the school system?

Again, that varies from child to child. My son needed speech therapy to learn how to start and maintain a conversation, how to determine what the other person is saying, how to listen to the other person and how to talk about something other than whatever his main focus was at that moment. In other words, when Josh was 7 years old, he needed help with social speech, rather than simply forming words or sentences. He knew how to talk, and did so beautifully, and would discourse for hours on Mighty Morphin Power Rangers or some other topic with no thought whatsoever about whether the other person in the conversation was the least bit interested. At first we got some pretty strange looks when we asked for speech therapy, but we demonstrated how it would help him, and luckily the speech and language therapist in our system understood what was necessary, and championed our request.

Your child might not need speech therapy. Instead, he might need social skills training, something our school system did not offer in the mid-1990s. Or, he might need language therapy and social skills training. Or he might need some other type of service.

Many children on the spectrum, including my son, need occupational therapy to help with the fine-motor skills delays that are quite common in spectrum disorders. Josh had OT for a number of years in school, and while he's never going to be the most dexterous person who ever lived, his handwriting is pretty legible, and he draws cartoons freehand, something we don't believe he would have been able to do without the therapy.

Other therapies, including applied behavioral analysis (ABA), a treatment that uses principles of behavioral therapy to change autistic "behaviors," are sometimes indicated for children on the spectrum. If your child is young enough (at 16, ABA might not make much of a difference to my son, but that doesn't mean it won't for your teenager) and a professional has indicated that ABA or other therapies (such as "brushing," for example, a therapy that uses a soft brush applied on the arms, legs and back to make the person feel less stressed by touch, etc.) might help, you will have to make your case to the school system when you attend an IEP meeting and work out the necessary services.

Knowing what to ask for is a tricky proposition in and of itself. Sometimes, it's best to consult with a psychologist, a pediatric neurologist or an educational specialist outside the school system before you begin to request services from the school. Analyze your child's strengths and weaknesses, determine what abilities need some improvement, and what therapies or techniques are necessary to achieve those improvements.

It's not necessary to consult an advocate at this point, as you're not yet involved in negotiating with the school. Rather, you're planning by creating a list of the services you think are necessary for your child, not a "wish list" of services you think would be nice, but that aren't essential to her having a successful school career.

When you're clear ahead of time on this issue, when you have specific knowledge of your child's needs and the services you think can help her, you can walk into an IEP meeting with a degree of confidence, and confidence means you don't have to go in with Guns A' Blazing. By preparing ahead of time, you'll not only have a clear idea of the services you think your child should have, you'll also have a store of knowledge that can help illustrate your point and bolster your chances of getting exactly what your child needs.

But again, it's important to go in with your ears open. If you have decided that a certain therapy is important to your child's education and the school district offers something else, that doesn't automatically mean battle lines must be drawn. It's possible the suggestion being made by the school is as good or better than the service you're requesting. Listen and then decide. You don't have to sign the IEP until it meets with your approval, and indeed, you shouldn't sign it until all the language it includes is what you believe your child should experience in school.

But remember the old saw about being careful what you ask for. One New York City couple told me their son was evaluated while in preschool, and his IEP included things the parents had never requested. "I was expecting to have to fight to get (my son) services," his mother says. "Instead, they were trying to pile on more than he needed." Leery of having her son pulled out of class too often, she requested that some of the services be scaled back and, eventually, the situation was corrected. But that story is the exception, and not the rule.

Most of the parents I spoke to for this book were concerned that the school system hadn't offered adequate supports or services for their children, and therefore had gone to various lengths to acquire what they thought was necessary. In some cases, the dispute between what the school saw as adequate and what the parents thought was essential ended up in a due process hearing, a mediation or a series of increasingly unpleasant phone calls and letters back and forth. In other instances, parents withdrew their children from the school, requested an out-of-district placement, asked for a transfer to another school or another class within the district or decided to go the route of home schooling.

It would be unfair to say that all the parents who did not feel their children's services were sufficient would have "done better" in their dealings with schools had they merely prepared their requests sooner or more completely. But there are some instances in which that was the case.

"I've seen parents come in and ask for the moon," one teacher in Pennsylvania told me. "They think that the school is obligated to provide the best in everything to every student, and that's not true. We're required to provide adequate services, enough to give the child the same education as everyone else. And I've never seen a case where the teachers and the school didn't want to do that."

It's a natural urge to want to provide the best for your child – our one serious point of contention with our school system so far involved sending our son to a special needs day camp during the summer at a cost of $1,000 a week. But it's necessary to be realistic when we're dealing with schools. Are there services you think would benefit your child, but that he doesn't really need? It might be best to foot the bill for those yourself. If finances are a problem, it's feasible to request extra services from the school, and maybe you'll get lucky. But don't expect it to be automatic, or easy.

If you "pad" your list with requests you're relatively sure will be rejected, you might think you're increasing the chances that you'll receive at least the items on your list that you consider essential. However, that is not always the case. The Pennsylvania teacher told me that "in some cases, you can tell when a parent is asking for something so they can get something else. But sometimes that just antagonizes everybody. We're still interested in giving each child what they need, but the meeting will take a much less friendly tone from there."

Making close personal friends is not the goal of an IEP meeting, and sometimes it is necessary to go to the mat over something your child really needs. But that should be a last resort, not a first, as it will color all future encounters between you and the people with whom your child spends a very large portion of his day.

Make a list of the services and supports you believe your child needs. And if you like, add the things you hope he could have, but that he can get by without. Request what you think is reasonable, and listen to the suggestions offered. You might be surprised that others have ideas that fit your child's academic profile better than what you are requesting. Remember, these people spend a lot of time in school with your child. It's possible they know a few things about him. If not, it's time for the guns to blaze.

Prior planning is important to all things on the autism spectrum – you've already discovered that, no doubt. And when you're getting ready to plan your child's school year, it feels like every detail is going to be enormous.

Relax. The important things will be obvious once you sit down and think about your child's personality and the nature of his spectrum disorder. Yes, it would be nice to add services that will make his life easier, and you should try to do that. But if you end up coming away from the meeting without the "luxuries," but with the "essentials," you have achieved your major goal. You should take yourself out to dinner and order a bottle of wine to celebrate.

Chapter Seven

IEP? INTERNATIONAL ELEPHANT PATROL?

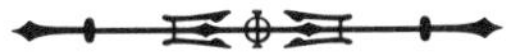

Frequently, we parents involved in the autism spectrum have conversations that sound like those of employees of Pentium discussing the best way to develop a new, faster information processing chip.

"I had to fight with my SD on the IEP to get OT, ST and a 1:1 for my son with PDD-NOS and ADHD."

"Ha! That's nothing. My daughter has HFA, or AS. I went to the IEP for ST and couldn't even get OT. And SST? They wouldn't even discuss it."

"You want to talk about ABA?"

"Pleeeeeeeeeeeease."

The alphabet soup makes sense to those of us who have been involved for a while, but at the beginning, well, it's alphabet soup.

The first acronym most of us learn is the one we deal with once a year or more often: the IEP. The Individualized Education Plan is, to give the most literal definition, a tool devised by parents, teachers and school personnel to define and describe the needs of the child and any special accommodations that are necessary to provide the child with whatever he needs to get the same education as everyone else in the school, if such a thing is possible.

The IEP is, without question, the point of contention most often brought up between parents and school systems about children on the spectrum. A well-written (and implemented) IEP can be a shining example of what can happen when a child with an autism spectrum disorder is given the proper evaluation and offered the kinds of accommodations necessary to help him thrive. On the other hand, an IEP that is put together with clenched teeth, between a school system that wants to save its pennies by cutting any "unnecessary" expenditure and a family desperate to get nothing but "the best" for a child, can be a document that is doomed to failure and misinterpretation. Even a good IEP can be destroyed by bad implementation.

In my son's case, the IEP has been a helpful, if flawed, tool. Our minor difficulties have come more often from teachers who haven't read the document rather than the IEP document itself. Usually, the IEP meetings we hold annually with teachers, administrators and, lately, Josh himself, have been very pleasant, often instructive to me about new possibilities, and almost never adversarial or contentious. Almost never.

There was one year when, after spending a number of summers (and a great deal of money we were hard pressed to find) sending him to a special needs summer camp, we asked the school district to grant Josh the status of an extended school year (ESY, if you love acronyms). This type of accommodation is meant to help children who, because of their specific disorder, have difficulty with the summer break – they tend to have fallen further behind than other children when the new school year opens, and take longer to catch up. While Josh's academics are very good, he does have trouble starting a new school year, and that is when his social issues related to his Asperger Syndrome are most evident. He gets himself into more "incidents" in September and October than any other months of the school year, and his grades in the first marking period are traditionally his lowest of the year. He spends the rest of the term catching up, and always raises his grades to their traditional level by June.

Then, the summer starts again.

In requesting extended school year, we were hoping the school district would agree that the program Josh had been attending, a special needs day camp geared toward children with AS, high-functioning autism and related disorders, was the best possible option to help him smooth out his school year and start the new term with a fresh perspective and a better chance to pick up where he had left his schoolwork 10 weeks earlier. And the school system agreed.

That is, it agreed that the camp was the best possible option. It did not agree that the best possible option was necessary and appropriate in Josh's case. The administrators, who had been resistant to the concept of an extended school year to begin with, did come around to the idea that it could help our son, but they were offering the school system's own summer program. However, we felt that, as described, it was appropriate for children with learning disabilities, emotional issues or academic problems, none of which described Joshua.

Needless to say, that IEP meeting did not go as smoothly and pleasantly as the others.

While it never became acrimonious, the meeting did illustrate for me the type of disagreements that parents often tell me about when discussing their children's IEP meetings. Tiny points can be argued about, important issues can be ignored in favor of minutia, and the main goal – helping the child – can become secondary to the sort of psychodrama that goes into any interaction between human beings who disagree. Passion can sometimes overshadow reason, on both sides of the table, and the end result is something less than what everyone set out to do at the beginning.

WHAT BELONGS IN AN IEP?

An IEP is not a biography of your child. It will include some information about his diagnosis and how it was reached (more on the ways the disorder manifests itself), but mostly, it will touch upon several areas in which some accommodations might be made and some help offered. These can include (but are by no means limited to):

1. An aide (paraprofessional or otherwise), who will be assigned to your child's case, and help him through the rough spots in the day, keep him focused on his work and help with organization;
2. An assignment to a "team teaching" class in which there is an extra teacher in the room, not necessarily assigned to your child, but with knowledge of your child's case and what problems may arise;
3. Any therapies (occupational, speech and language, etc.) that might be required and the protocols for them, including whether your child is removed from class to receive therapy, or if it is done during non-school hours;
4. Any accommodations needed to best measure your child's academic progress (extra time on tests, a computer to type, rather than write, answers, etc.);
5. Plans to help your child avoid difficult situations, and to deal with any particularly troublesome areas (phobias, sensory sensitivities, social skills difficulties, etc.).

That's just the beginning of a good IEP. Beyond that should come very specialized, individually considered and designed plans for academic success as well as social growth and progress maturing emotionally. For children who need special therapies such as ABA, for example, these may – or may not – be specified in the IEP. Children who need help in one class can have this specified in the IEP. For example, at one point, my son needed certain parts of his French tests to be repeated for him.

The key is this: Any concern you have about your child that relates to his or her disorder can and should be addressed in the IEP. It doesn't matter how specific it is to your child, or even if your child is the only person on the planet to whom this might apply. If it will help to make an accommodation, and that accommodation is reasonably available within the school system, it should at least be considered for inclusion in his IEP.

Consider, as well, that just because something is included in an IEP doesn't mean you ever have to use it. For years, we asked for an accommodation that Josh be given seating preference in his classes, specifying that he should be seated near the teacher, at the front of the room, whenever possible. This was because when he was a small boy it made him more comfortable if he could see and hear everything that went on, and frankly, because it usually meant one fewer of his peers would be sitting adjacent to his desk, possibly teasing him. We still have that provision in his IEP, even though we haven't asked for it to be implemented in years. Josh, now about 5'10", does not need to be seated in the front of the classroom in order to see the board.

Similarly, when it was decided, after a number of years, that Josh no longer needed the occupational therapy he had been given, we asked that the possibility to begin the OT again be written into the IEP, just in case we saw his handwriting or fine-motor skills erode. We haven't had to ask for more OT, but we keep it in the IEP, so we know it will be available if it becomes necessary.

Parents are extremely wary, and should be, of conceding any accommodation if they don't know it can be replaced or revived should the need arise. An IEP offers the "security blanket" of leaving the options open, so that any necessary accommodation can be implemented immediately if needed.

If the IEP meeting doesn't go the way parents hope it will, we have an option: We can refuse to sign the completed document. But be careful. When you attend the IEP meeting at school, you'll be asked (in most states) to sign a form that indicates you were in attendance. That is not the same as signing the IEP. If you do attend the meeting, you should certainly sign the form that says you attended.

But if the IEP that is written at the meeting does not include provisions you think are essential, or includes provisions you think could be detrimental to your child, you don't have to sign the final document. In fact, you shouldn't sign the final document if you disagree with anything it contains.

When one Missouri woman found that her school district wanted to place her son in a special education classroom and she thought it was inappropriate, "I learned the power of the IEP," she says. She refused to sign the document, and wrote a letter specifying precisely why she would not sign it in its current form. "The withholding of your signature on that document causes all kinds of things to happen," she says. "I was nice, but I was persistent. Somebody at the district level saw that there was no IEP in place and that they were implementing changes anyway, and suddenly they were caught." Things changed quickly, and her son remained in an included classroom.

It's important to learn the rules that govern your state's (or country's) rules regarding an IEP. Where I live, as with many states, the regulations are specific, but they can be misleading. If I disagree with the wording or content of my son's IEP, I don't have to sign it. But I must express – in writing – my objections to the IEP within 15 days of receiving the final copy, or the IEP will be implemented whether I object or not. This is *not* true of a first IEP, which requires that the guardian's signature be implemented, but of all subsequent versions. So be sure to make the source of your displeasure known, and be sure to keep copies for anyone who might have questions later on.

Also, once the IEP is in place, it's vital that it be implemented properly. That means you have to be more vigilant than ever after you have participated in the process of developing the plan. Make sure every teacher who will interact with your child has a copy of the completed IEP. And make sure they read it. Speak to each one at the beginning of the term and ask if they have any questions. Make sure you reiterate any specific concerns you have – even if they are addressed in the IEP. Write a letter with the answer to any teacher who had a question and refer to the IEP. Keep a copy.

I have never needed to use any of the copies of the letters I've made, and yet I continue to make them. I talk to the teachers at the beginning of every school year, even if I wait until Back to School Night to do so. I make sure they've read Josh's IEP and understand what it says. And I have a strong backup, in that his classroom aide, Mrs. Gregus, is in school every day, and I know for a fact that she has read the IEP – she was at the meeting where it was written.

Chapter Eight

PARAPROFESSIONALS DON'T JUMP OUT OF AIRPLANES

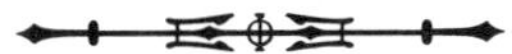

An "aide." A "helper." A "one-on-one." A "classroom aide." No matter what he or she is called, the most personal, constant type of assistance for a child on the autism spectrum is a full-time aide, a person who assists in the classroom (and the hallways, and the gymnasium, and the lunchroom ...) when the "rough spots" of the day, like paying attention in class, getting through lunch without being teased or just getting through physical education can be more difficult than for neurotypical children.

When it works well, the relationship between a child with a neurological condition or impairment and a classroom aide can be the most helpful type of accommodation – it benefits the child, the teacher, the class and the school (in that order) in ways that can't be measured, but are undeniably valuable. When it doesn't work well, it can be the therapeutic equivalent of fingernails on a blackboard.

It's a very personal, very specific type of chemistry that goes on between the aide (sometimes a paraprofessional and sometimes an untrained aide, occasionally someone with training in special education) and the student. There were times when Mrs. Gregus was my son's closest friend in school in his younger days. There were also times when he would have preferred to go through his day on his own.

Every year, the IEP meeting would begin with the question of an aide. When Josh was in second grade, there was no question: He needed the individual help that a devoted paraprofessional could deliver, and once he met Mrs. Gregus in third grade, there was no question as to who that staff member should be. But as he grew older, and needed more independence, it wasn't Mrs. Gregus' devotion or skill that was in question; it was Josh's need for an aide at all.

Joyce became the stable force in his school day, and my wife and I would find reasons that she could not be reassigned: This would be a transition year from one school to another; Josh was starting middle school; next year, he'd be starting high school, and the transition would be too difficult without his human safety net.

As I write this, we are struggling with the question again.

It's just becoming spring, and the annual IEP meeting for Josh will be held in the next six weeks. We'll discuss his progress this year (good, but not without its rough days), his transition plans after high school (he wants to go to a four-year college; mostly because that's what we've told him he wants) and what his course load for next year should look like (if we have our way, it will consist of all honors classes, but that's a story for another chapter).

Then, there will be the question about Mrs. Gregus. I have no idea how I'm going to answer it. By the time you read this, I will know, but that doesn't help me all that much right now.

On the one hand, there's the "don't-mess-with-success" theory, which essentially states that if the student has been succeeding the way things are, it would be crazy to disrupt the situation, especially in such a basic way as taking away his main line of support. There's no point in making him deal with things that are especially difficult for him, particularly as he's trying to maintain a grade point average that will help him with admission to colleges and to establish a more complete social life at the same time, never an easy task for an Asperger kid.

However, there's the other hand, too: Josh is 15 years old, and at some point he will have to deal with the world independently. In college, a mere three years from now, there will probably not be someone organizing his notes, compiling his homework assignments and keeping him out of the way of people who might irritate him to the point that he would act inappropriately. Mrs. Gregus, for all our joking about her rooming with Josh in college, will not be there in three years. Shouldn't we find out now how he'll react, while there's still time to prepare him better?

Finally, no matter how beloved or effective an aide is, a high school sophomore being trailed by a middle-aged woman is not likely to be at the center of the social scene. There will be talk, there will be giggling, and there will be an arm's length between Josh and almost all the other teens in his classes. That, for a child on the autism spectrum, is not a small consideration.

The most worrisome aspect of an IEP for a parent is the idea that if you give up an accommodation, a therapy or an aide, it will be difficult, if not impossible, to get it back in future IEPs or in mid-year, should the student hit a rough spot.

One thing is practically certain: If we don't request an aide in next year's IEP, and Josh has difficulty coping without one, even if the school district agrees to replace her, the person dealing with him next year will not be Joyce Gregus.

After seven years, that's not an easy thing to write.

Some parents believe that a personal aide (a "one-on-one" or 1:1 in the current jargon) is not a good idea anyway. They think that the constant presence of an adult whose job it is to "guide" the student through a day at school is in itself enough to alienate classmates or to invite teasing. They also believe that the student will not develop independence if there is always an adult at his side to help him through the rough spots.

There is an argument to be made in that area, but I know that in third or fourth grade, my son would have had a very difficult time if he had not had that support. That's one case. Others point to another conclusion.

Again, this is an area in which you know your own child better than anyone else. If you truly believe that your child can get through a typical school day, make the decisions, deal with the situations and the people, and be able to get everything done that his peers do every day, without a paraprofessional, that is probably the way to go. The least restriction, the least inhibition, the better in many cases. But if getting through an "average" day is more than your child can handle, and the attention of another adult would help get him through the challenges that other children handle instinctively, it might be best to request, and fight for, an aide in the classroom.

This can be accomplished in one of two ways. The one-on-one aide, who is assigned to one student and whose primary responsibility is to that student, is considered a "luxury" by many school systems, particularly those whose budgets are especially limited. And some parents, as noted above, believe the extra attention brought by an aide can be detrimental to the student's social growth. An alternative is the "classroom aide," a paraprofessional (usually this term implies a certain amount of training, but that may or may not be present) whose responsibility is to several students in the class, and who acts primarily as an adjunct to the main classroom teacher.

This idea works for some parents and students, the theory being that there is support when needed, but without the "stigma" of a full-time aide whose presence makes the student seem more "different" than necessary.

Some students require a level of support that cannot be accomplished by a classroom aide who must divide his or her attention among all the students in the class. When a child starts to feel stressed and must leave the classroom, for example, it is more difficult for a classroom aide to escort him into the hallway and discuss the situation to rectify it and move on.

Sometimes a "shadow aide," or one who goes to great lengths to "hang back" and intervene only when necessary, is the best solution. This type of support is as non-intrusive as the student's needs allow, thereby making it easier for other children to approach without fear of being watched by "a teacher."

One New York parent told me her son "had a fabulous shadow" in his preschool class, but early intervention had made a huge difference in his work, and now the aide was no longer needed. "He's now getting 12 hours of ABA therapy a week, and I can't imagine how much money (the district) is spending on my kid," she says. "It's a giant poster for early intervention. They took a chance, and they're creating a functioning child."

Many of the parents I interviewed would have been delighted to have a one-on-one aide assigned to their children, but could not convince their school systems such a move was necessary. "It's all about money," one Nebraska mom told me. "They can see (my son) needs the help, but they're pretending they don't see it because they can't afford the extra staff."

Of course, a school system will never tell a parent that a service can't be included in an IEP because of budgetary restraints, since they are required by law to provide the necessary accommodations regardless of their budget. And as one father pointed out to me, "they're going to get state or federal money if they need it, and that's never the point. It's that they don't want to spend the money on one child, but they're required to."

For children on the spectrum, for whom organization is a huge issue, the "safety net" of a paraprofessional, particularly one who is trained in autism spectrum disorders, can be invaluable. In some cases, it is an absolute necessity. But when a school system refuses to acknowledge the need for extra help, parents and school systems often cross the line into a Guns A' Blazing situation.

In our son's case, the help he has gotten for the past seven years has been absolutely central to his growth and development. As parents, we are certain he would not have performed as well academically or progressed as far socially as he has if he had not been able to relax and stop worrying about the stressful situations that Mrs. Gregus helped him manage. His skills in dealing with those situations has grown as well, since he's seen, over a long period of time, that they can be handled, and are not insurmountable obstacles.

When necessary, Joyce has learned to "hang back" and give Joshua his space. She knows that he needs to feel independent, and be able to interact with peers without her visible presence. Given that, she sometimes performs tasks at a teacher's request that take her out of the classroom for periods of time. For example, she has a lunch break during one of Josh's classes and, therefore, is not present. She's helped him through some rough spots, but she's let him handle a few himself as well. It hasn't been easy for her, as she's very protective of Josh, but she knows, as a parent does, that he has to grow, and doing everything for him isn't going to help him do that.

Whether it's this year or next, it won't be easy to say goodbye. In my son's case, the relationship has been a very successful one indeed.

Thank you, Joyce.

Chapter Nine

THE LESS SQUEAKY WHEEL GETS THE GOOD BAGELS

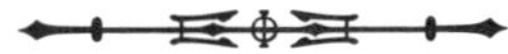

There is no discounting the horror stories – they're true, they're disturbing, and they offer a cautionary tale to any of us with children on the autism spectrum. However, they're not the only stories.

In fact, it's not a stretch of the imagination to say that the vast majority of parents with "special needs" children have a perfectly workable relationship with their school systems. They meet regularly, discuss options, agree (or compromise) on services and stay focused on the fact that their common goal is to help the student.

No, it's not a fairy tale. It's just that this isn't the kind of experience you're used to hearing about. Yet, it's the kind that happens most of the time.

When we first hear the "autism" word, we're scared. And among the very things we do is to seek out other parents who have had or are having similar experiences, if for no other reason than to commiserate. If you can't complain to someone who's likely to understand, you feel more alone and more isolated. There's enough stress already.

When we discover other parents with similar experiences, it's likely to be through one of two avenues: friends of someone we know who have a child on the spectrum, or parents who belong to a support group, one that we discover and decide to join. These are special places, relationships we will treasure for the rest of our lives, in some cases.

The first time I attended a meeting of ASPEN, the group then just being organized by Lori Shery and others in Edison, New Jersey, I didn't know what to expect. I'm not the type who joins groups much; freelance writers work by themselves in our homes and are, generally speaking, the modern equivalent of hermits, dealing with our families and a few close friends (met before we began freelancing, when we had ties to the outside world). I wasn't sure what I expected to get from the meeting, but I thought there might be some information I could use to help my (then) 5-year-old son as he started school.

But I found immediate benefits beyond information. For one thing, as people began to share their experiences, I realized that maybe I wasn't the worst parent in the world, which was a concern of mine at the time. I heard them tell their stories, and I related to them. I understood that we all have a difficult path to take, and the fact that others were reacting the same way I did made me feel a little bit more secure. I made friends with a few, listened to others, and after a few meetings, became bold enough to tell my stories, too.

Still, there was something that bothered me: Everyone there seemed to have had some awful, nightmarish experience with their child's school and the people who worked there. As Josh was just finishing his year in kindergarten, and the Child Study Team was completing their testing on him at the time, this was very disturbing news, indeed.

All these people whose experiences seemed so close to mine were having hideous trials and tribulations with schools. Didn't that, by extension, mean that I'd be having the same torturous problems some time soon? How could Josh get through his school years (and this strange Transitional Primary year the school was proposing) if the teachers and administrators I met were more concerned with clearing him off their budget than giving him the accommodations he needed?

Luckily, I am married to a very level-headed woman, and after we talked at length, we agreed that our school system was, indeed, doing what it could – and what was necessary – for our son. We followed the advice the Child Study Team was giving us, added some concerns of our own, which they accepted willingly, and his IEP was in place before he began the next year at school. Cooler heads prevailed.

Since then, we have rarely had a major disagreement with our school system and its representatives; yet there have been a few bumps along the way. But we've learned that we can't always assume an issue will go well or badly based on what other parents' experiences have been. We have to trust our own judgment, get the best information we can, and make a choice.

Sometimes, I think we parents do others a disservice when we emphasize the difficulties we've had helping our children with autism or another spectrum disorder through school. Yes, we should warn those who don't have our level of experience as to what the problems may be. Yes, we should vent our spleens when something hideous is done to our children in the name of education, and we shouldn't stop complaining until the wrong is made right. Absolutely, we need to make as much of a fuss as is necessary, and to get as much attention paid to the disorders our children face, to better help "normal" children and their parents understand why our children might not act the way they expect. But, we shouldn't be telling "rookies" that the only possible school experience is a negative one.

Because it's not.

When my wife and I attended one of Josh's IEP meetings a few years ago, it was early in the morning (so my wife could get to work as soon as possible). We knew there weren't many major issues to settle, but we had concerns and questions, and we expected to meet with some concerns and questions from the Child Study Team as well. Josh had been having a good year at school, but there were the usual challenges along the way, and they needed to be addressed as the next year's plan was being considered.

We came into the conference room (which was actually the school social worker's office), and were just sitting down when the school psychologist arrived. She asked if we'd like something to eat; they had brought in bagels and muffins from a local bakery and had brewed a fresh pot of coffee because it was the first meeting of the morning.

We knew there were others who did not always get along with the Child Study Team, and we knew that some of them had legitimate reasons to have grievances. But we'd had a smooth relationship with almost everyone attending the meeting this morning. I looked over at the school psychologist, told her I was going to go without breakfast that morning (I usually do), and thanked her. She smiled at me.

"But we knew you were coming in first this morning," she joked. "We got the good bagels."

Sometimes, the less squeaky wheels get the good bagels.

Now, I'm not for a moment advocating that parents whose children have legitimate needs for special services should simply acquiesce whenever a school system says to, simply to get better pastry at an IEP meeting. I'm not saying you should give even an inch in your requests for necessary services just to get the people who work at the school to like you. If your child needs some help, and the school doesn't want to provide it, you need to fight tooth and nail, by all means necessary, until that accommodation is made. Period.

However, we also need to keep an eye on what is reasonable. We don't have the right to request a better education for our children, but we have every right to demand an equal education, and for our children, "equal" might require some extraordinary means. That's okay, and if that's what they need, we should be sure our children receive it.

However, we should wait for the school to be unreasonable before we start pulling out the heavy artillery.

When you meet someone for the first time, you don't immediately assume that person is a psychopathic serial murderer, even if you have seen plenty of movies about psychopathic serial murderers who appeared to be "normal" until they committed their hideous crimes. You don't take it for granted that all people who dress a certain way are going to attack you in the street. You don't guess that people who come from a certain state are bad drivers. Even if your friends say they didn't like a particular movie, you might go see it anyway, if the story appeals to you.

Similarly, there's no reason to think that because other parents whose children are on the autism spectrum have had bad experiences with schools that you will, too. If the parents aren't people from the same school district, dealing with the same teachers, administrators and support personnel, and if they aren't asking for the same accommodations for the same disorders, you can't extrapolate their experiences to yours.

Certainly, there are patterns. Some school districts get a bad reputation among parents for a reason. If the same stories about the same people under the same conditions are repeated enough times, you have to assume that where there's smoke, there's fire.

But you still need to wait for that behavior to be exhibited to you before you can assume it exists. You have to go into the first meeting with the stories you've heard filed away, assuming that the school system is prepared to be reasonable and helpful, and then accept it if the people you talk to are, in fact, reasonable and helpful.

Too many parents go to meetings assuming things will be bad, and they begin by behaving as if the school system has already refused their children essential services. If you react to reputation, to the horror stories you've heard (true or not) before you see evidence in your own child's case, you're asking for trouble. No, you're demanding trouble.

Yet, parents who tell horror stories do a lot of good sometimes. They can warn parents whose children are newly diagnosed about the problems that can arise; they can help you learn what to ask for. They can illustrate the difficulty we sometimes go through just to level the playing field for our children. They undeniably help simply by telling their stories and letting us know that it's not always going to be easy.

But when we hear those stories and make the mental leap to the conclusion that because it happened to them, it will happen to us, we're not reacting well. We're not doing the best we can for our children and we're not doing ourselves a favor either. We're paving the road to the services our children need, and we're paving it with land mines.

Take every anecdote (even the ones in this book), good and bad, with a grain of salt. Absorb the information, assume it's true, but don't immediately decide that your experience will, by definition, be the same, because it's possible, if not probable, that it won't be. Your experience with a school system will be colored by any number of variables – your personality, the personalities of those working in the school system, the state you live in (or the country you live in), the disorder your child has, its severity, the accommodations your child needs, and many, many others – that can't possibly be the same as those of the people telling you their horror story.

My experience has been that if you treat education professionals in a reasonable manner, they will respond in a reasonable manner. If you try to see things through their eyes, you should find common ground. And if you really and truly believe your child needs a certain service, you can usually find a way to get it.

But that's just my experience. It may not be yours. I can't guarantee, even to people who live in the same school district that I do, that they won't be telling someone else a horror story one year from now. What I know is, the less squeaky wheels sometimes get the good bagels.

Chapter Ten

AUTISM SPECTRUM PARENTS, UNITE!

You can tell the "rookies" at the support group meetings. They're the ones with the "deer-in-the-headlights" glare in their eyes, the slightly tremulous lower lip, the bend to the neck that makes them spend time staring at their shoes. They don't stick out like a sore thumb, but they are easy to identify.

It's understandable. Most newcomers to parent support groups are people whose children (grandchildren, nephews, nieces, friends) have been very recently diagnosed. They're still reeling from the news, perhaps just shaking off the last traces of denial, and wondering if coming to this room, with these people, was really a good move. They know they've been miserable failures as parents, and feel that fact is certain to show among these paragons of patience, sanity and wisdom.

Then, they hear their first exchange. Parents complaining about the miserable way teachers are treating their children. Confessing that they sometimes feel inadequate to the task of raising a child with special needs. Wondering aloud if they're doing everything they can do to help, and if not, what else there is to try. Saying what most of us think, but don't always have the courage to express out loud: I'm just making this up as I go along – I could be making awful mistakes.

Suddenly, the "rookies" lose that terrified look. They begin to nod their heads. They make more frequent eye contact. They might even – if they think no one is looking – risk a smile, albeit a small one. They're starting to get the message: "We're all in the same boat. Welcome, and here's your oar."

There is strength in numbers, and the work of an autism spectrum parent is something that can't necessarily be done by one or two people alone. We need to band together, to recognize that others are experiencing what we go through on a daily basis, and that there are ways to make the job a little easier, if not actually easy. The mental, psychological burden might be just a touch lighter when we come to terms with the fact that there are others much like us.

New parents who find comrades in arms for the first time look so unburdened that their whole demeanor changes. Some make friends they will keep for life. Others simply absorb the information that's given, perhaps contribute some experiences of their own, and then move on, strengthened by the knowledge that there are people out there who have the same concerns and can offer a few solutions.

My belief is that few things are more essential to parents whose child is on the spectrum than the realization that they are not alone. It can start off feeling like such a singular, isolated experience (especially if one is a single parent, or if one's spouse is not on board with the program immediately) that just seeing the friendly faces and hearing similar-sounding experiences in one place can be something of a revelation in itself.

When we're dealing with school systems, however, it's a double-edged sword. There's good and bad to the shared experience, but the good far outweighs its counterpart.

First of all, it's important to know that there are others in the same school system who have similar concerns. Yours is not the first child to come to this school with an autism spectrum disorder, no matter how surprised or ill informed the teachers and administrators seem to be on the subject. So understanding that point is a step in the right direction.

By law, the school can't release the names of children who are classified with autism spectrum disorders (or anything else, for that matter) to the public. But it shouldn't be hard to find out who some of the children with similar challenges in your school district are, either from your own children, who would probably be able to identify those whose behavior is similar to theirs, or from other parents. The best way is to network within the spectrum.

"I had no idea there were other children with Asperger in my district," one mother from North Dakota told me. "The way the school was talking, I would have sworn (my son) was the first."

She decided to get on the Internet and check out a few Asperger-related chat rooms and bulletin boards. Sure enough, there were other parents in her area who were happy to share their experiences. One mom had a child in the same district, and they compared notes on which teachers were more sensitive to spectrum disorders and what had worked to help get services that were otherwise being held back by the school system. While the first mom has never met the second one to this day, they have supported each other through a difficult time and helped their children succeed more thoroughly in school.

"When I put out a (bulletin board post) asking about parents in North Dakota, I never expected to find one in my own district," she says. "That was just icing on the cake. But it proved to be really helpful. We managed to avoid one teacher who is really rigid and doesn't understand Asperger at all."

Local support groups that meet in person on a regular basis are invaluable, but in some remote areas, parents are scattered a bit more, and it's difficult to organize in a meaningful fashion. That is why the powers that be invented the Internet.

While I'll make no specific recommendations for chat rooms or bulletin boards, I can tell you that a recent Google search with the key words "Asperger," "autism" and "chat room" yielded no fewer than 105,000 sites to explore. With that kind of volume, it can be expected that sites provide every point of view on the subject, from those searching for a cure to those who disdain the very word "cure" and consider autism a personality type that society would do well to recognize and celebrate.

No matter where you fall on the issues, there is a place for you on the Internet. The key is to get on, find out what others are saying, and when you feel comfortable, join in the conversation. Make sure to check the rules of each bulletin board or list and adhere closely to them – many have forbidden topics, things that have come up too many times before or have proven a sore spot for members. Avoid those at all costs.

Getting the main points of view available, just finding out what sources of information exist, is enough of an advantage to make Internet support groups worthwhile. But the feeling of belonging, of being part of a group, is an even more satisfying benefit for many parents. Parenting children on the spectrum can be a lonely task, and merely discovering that others are going through the same trials as you are can make a difference. As you sit in front of your computer screen, imagine all those nodding heads at a real-time, in-person support group meeting when common experiences are shared.

But learning about programs and studies, and meeting other parents, is just the beginning. Whether online or in person, there can be strength in numbers for parents whose children need additional help. When a school system has achieved a negative reputation, it is possible to discover, through interaction with others, whether it is deserved, and where the problem might lie.

It's also possible, when other parents on the spectrum are in your area geographically, to act together in an attempt to get better services generally for children with autism spectrum disorders. Parents who appeal to administrators and school boards en masse have a better chance of being heard, and being taken seriously, than those who speak individually.

It's not necessary to "storm the Bastille" for every service you believe your child needs. It's not even necessary to go to the school superintendent or the elected board when one child or two have a problem that isn't being addressed. Those situations can usually be handled in smaller meetings, between parents and school personnel, and can progress naturally up the line from teacher to administrator to principal to superintendent, and so on, as is necessary.

When a school system (and this does occasionally happen) refuses to acknowledge children with autism spectrum disorders, assumes they are "behavior problems" or have a "mental illness," it can be very helpful to confront the entire system (after all other measures have been exhausted) with the strength in numbers of area parents. This does not have to be limited to parents whose children have autism spectrum disorders. Anyone whose child has a special need that isn't being met by the local system may be invited to participate.

Begin by stating the problem. No matter what, don't let the conversation get personal. This is not about you, and it's not about the teacher, principal, administrator or anyone else in the school system who may not be sensitive to autism spectrum disorders. It's about the children who need help, and how best to obtain it for them. And it is about all those children, not just yours or those of people you know. If the situation is that localized, there is no place for it in an open meeting – it can go to mediation or a due process hearing, if necessary.

Once the problem has been identified, you can suggest solutions. If the system is open to programs like ABA or something that requires outside help, you can begin by suggesting those things. If the system has not responded in the past, it's necessary to educate those involved about advances in therapies and programs that have proven to be effective in many cases.

Education is always the goal. No one therapy or program is perfect for every child on the spectrum, let alone every child with a special need in the district. What's important is to make sure the system knows the nature of the disorder in question, and what has proven effective to help the children who might need assistance. (While things are improving, I know from experience that the words "Asperger Syndrome" have not exactly entered the national lexicon, and in many cases are not recognized even by professionals who should have known about them more than 10 years ago.) Emphasize that the goal is not to provide more than other children in the system are entitled to, but to give children on the spectrum the same chance to get a complete education as every other child in the district.

Don't have one spokesperson. This leads to personal attacks and hurt feelings instead of progress and collective benefit. Make sure several members of the support group or parent's network are capable of speaking for the group, that virtually everyone is informed well enough to answer questions, and that a cool attitude and absolutely no words spoken in anger are the rules of the group.

Recruit parents of neurotypical children, too. This may sound difficult, but I'm willing to bet you have friends in the district (or school system) whose children fall into that category, and who would be willing to help. Stress that there will be benefits for all the children in the school, as less disruptive behavior and a more orderly learning environment are sure to result from treatments, therapies and better education.

There is strength in numbers, but being right doesn't hurt either. Don't dig in your heels and demand the moon when you know it's not possible, and in some cases, not fair. Don't lead a large group of parents into a battle you know you can't win. Choose your spots, only act as a group when it's necessary, and keep in mind:

You're not alone – that's something all by itself.

Chapter Eleven

DO I NEED AN ADVOCATE?

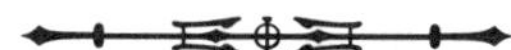

Most dealings between parents who have children on the autism spectrum and schools, either public or private, are just that. There are no third parties involved, and the parents tend to enter into such situations alone (for single parents, really alone).

In many situations, that's not a problem. When the school system and the parents agree on what is necessary and how to implement it, there's no need for anyone else to attend meetings, write letters or make phone calls on the parents' behalf. But as this book (and countless parents) will tell you, that isn't always the case.

In short, sometimes parents find that they can't handle the task alone. They need to know about school procedures, school district budgets and special education law, and they need to know all that while trying to get services for their children, hold down a job, pay the bills, cook dinner and maybe, once in a while, notice that there are people around other than a child who has an autism spectrum disorder. If it sounds overwhelming, it's only because that kind of life – common to many of us – can be exactly that – overwhelming.

Enter the advocate.

A parent advocate (actually an advocate for the child in question) is an independent, paid professional who consults with parents, helps determine what services are necessary, and then attends IEP meetings or other conferences with the school system to advocate on the parents' behalf. Quite often, they have come to the profession after experiencing these kinds of situations personally (many advocates have relatives or friends who are on the spectrum and know the difficulty school systems sometimes have with such children). They usually have a background in special education and a knowledge of the law in your state or country. And they are acquainted with therapies and services that are especially helpful for children with autism spectrum disorders.

But, how do you know if you need to contact an advocate? After all, they do charge a fee (which varies from state to state and advocate to advocate), which adds an expense to the list of those you're already handling. Some parents also feel strange about bringing an advocate to school meetings, believing it seems very much like a "Guns A' Blazing" tactic, and can make the proceedings seem more adversarial, rather than less.

"The best thing any parent can do if they're going to fight is never to go in alone," says one Colorado parent who has worked with an advocate. "If you write a letter and your district doesn't comply within 10 days, don't wait."

First of all, there is no reason for a parent to feel uncomfortable bringing an educational advocate or an attorney to any meeting with a school district. None. Ever. Even if you subscribe to the theory that you don't have to show up with your guns out of your holster until there's a reason to do so, you can still bring help immediately – before there's a problem. Bringing an advocate to a meeting in which you have every legal right to invite any person you please is not firing a shot across the school district's bow. It is leveling the playing field and making you feel more comfortable. If you think you might not be able to quote chapter and verse of your district's school budget and education law, and that you might need to, don't hesitate to seek the help of an advocate if you can afford the fee.

If you can't afford the fee, ask the advocate about ways to pay over time, or ways to finance that you might not have considered. Some parents take out loans, others can afford to pay the fee right away. Some advocates charge by the hour, others by the case. Get in touch with the local autism support groups and special education agencies to get information in your area.

If you have determined that you want to contact an advocate, how do you determine which advocate to contact? Do you need an advocate, or a lawyer?

"At the first sign of trouble with the district is the latest time to contact an attorney," says Ira Fingles, a partner in the law firm Hinkle and Fingles, a disability rights firm with offices in New Jersey and Pennsylvania. "There's no harm in contacting an attorney too early."

An attorney with a background in disability rights and special education law can be a great asset to parents facing an uncooperative school system. For one thing, once there is resistance from either side, a process begins that might end up in mediation, a due process hearing or even in court. Parents entering into that vortex without an attorney are asking for trouble, or at the very least, giving the school system the upper hand.

"A lot of school districts see a kid on the autism spectrum and start grinding for battle," Fingles says. "It's important for parents to be familiar with the procedures, but parents don't need to be that well steeped in the law. That's what the attorney is for."

Disputes can begin even at the prospect of an evaluation. Sometimes school districts don't believe a child needs to be evaluated by their Child Study Team when parents believe the child should. (Other times, it's the other way around.) Or parents and schools might disagree on who should do the testing. Some parents believe that specialists on the payroll of the school district are more likely to provide an evaluation that matches the district's opinion, rather than taking all the facts into account.

"The school district is obligated to ensure that whoever is doing the evaluation is qualified," Fingles says. "Parents must be satisfied with the credentials, and the school system has to be able to provide documentation."

One school administrator in New Jersey told me that "schools don't ask (specialists) for a particular diagnosis or classification. But sometimes, parents believe that the (specialist) is going to tell the school what it wants to hear. I've been in plenty of meetings where the expert didn't say what the school had been saying; I know that it happens."

No matter whether the dispute is real or imagined, an independent advocate in the room will argue on the parents' (and by extension, the child's) side, but that doesn't mean no advocate will ever recommend a compromise. Some parents really do expect more than their children are entitled to, and some school systems really are trying to provide the necessary accommodations, even when it appears they're not. It's the advocate's job to communicate what the parents see as the problem, suggest possible solutions, and help both sides come to a conclusion that will benefit the child.

When discussing a school district, I've spoken to too many parents who talk about what "I got" when dealing with schools, what "I needed" at a meeting and what "they did to me" to think that all parents with children on the spectrum are thinking only about what's right for their children. It gets personal, and when it gets personal, sometimes the overall goal – helping the child with the disorder – is lost in the process, a victim of the venom both sides are spewing. It can get ugly. Emotion can overcome reason in humans, and parents, teachers and school administrators are only human.

So are advocates, but they are not immediately involved in the situation. A good advocate knows how to defuse potentially explosive situations, and how to direct the discussion back to the purpose at hand. "I've seen letters that have gone back and forth between parents and school systems that border on the combative," one Pennsylvania-based advocate told me. "I've seen situations where ego and personalities got involved, and that never helps. If you think they're doing this just to get back at you for being a pain, you're at a disadvantage – even if you're right," she adds.

Once you've determined that a parent's advocate or an educational law attorney might be necessary in your child's case, how do you find a reputable one? Again, local and national support groups for parents of autism spectrum children can be helpful, either from their websites or by contacting them directly by phone. They often have lists of advocates and attorneys in local areas, or will be able to recommend a few for you to choose from.

When you call to discuss your child's situation, ask for references, parents of children on the spectrum for whom the advocate or attorney has worked before. Get their phone numbers, and call them up. Find out what the person's strengths and weaknesses are, and decide if they match the kind of assistance you're going to need. These people are professionals, and will not take it personally if you don't hire them because they're not right for the job.

Questions to ask include: Have you worked with this school system before? Have you worked with this particular disorder before? What do you need to know before we begin the process about my child? How do you envision this case proceeding? How much will it cost?

Make sure the questions are answered to your satisfaction, even if the answers aren't the ones you want to hear. Make sure you understand exactly what you're signing on for when you hire the advocate, because the last thing you want is to have to change to someone else while you're in the middle of talks with the district.

Make sure you find someone who has experience with your child's disorder, because the spectrum is, as you are well aware, not limited to one set of behaviors or one set of difficulties. It's best to have the advocate meet your child before you hire him or her, so the person who will be working with you has an idea of what your child needs.

Make sure that all records – every test, every evaluation, every diagnosis and every piece of correspondence between you and the school system – are made available to the advocate you choose. Your advocate doesn't want any surprises when it's time to discuss strategies, therapies and accommodations. Too much information is always better than not enough.

Let your school district know you're bringing an advocate to the meeting. There's no advantage in keeping that information to yourself, and it will make for a smoother session when the advocate is expected. But listen to the advocate's (or attorney's) advice on this subject, and then decide for yourself what makes sense.

In the interest of full disclosure, I must report that my wife and I have never felt the need to hire an advocate. My wife is an attorney, although not one with a background in special education law, and our dealings with the local school district have not come to the point that we felt an expert was needed. But if we do in the next few years (our son will be a high school senior in three years, as of this writing), we will not hesitate to seek out the necessary support.

I'll discuss the process of mediation, due process and the like later in this book. Suffice it here to say that when you hire an advocate, the process is less lonely, bolstered with someone who has the necessary experience and the facts at hand to help make your child's case for him. But hiring an advocate does not guarantee the outcome you desire, and the fee charged is not contingent on your child receiving the services or accommodations you outline at the beginning. An advocate is another bullet to put in that gun, but there are plenty of things that have to go right in order to make the shot hit the mark when you need it.

CHAPTER TWELVE

THE VORTEX – WHEN PARENTS AND SCHOOLS DISAGREE

Let's begin by noting that there's no such thing as the "one way" that a dispute between parents and a school system will proceed. Within countries, within states, sometimes within school districts, there can be variations. There can be differences between the laws from state to state. There can be variations in procedure. There can be differences as basic as those between two teachers who have contrasting styles. In other words, I cannot tell you exactly how your dispute will proceed, or how it will be settled.

Now that we've gotten the disclaimers out of the way, let's talk about how you can get pulled into The Vortex.

Of course, that's not something you want to do; it's best to avoid The Vortex when you can. In fact, it's only when the first line of defense – the "No Guns A' Blazing" approach – and the second – the "Guns A' Blazing" approach – fail that you should begin the steps that will pull you into The Vortex.

What is The Vortex? It's the process of challenges and legal proceedings that lead from quiet meetings in school buildings to not-so-quiet hearings in courtrooms. It is the way parents with children on the autism spectrum find themselves trying desperately to secure the fundamental, essential services and accommodations that go with the proper education of a child with an autism-related disorder.

Parents who have been there are the ones most likely to have horror stories, whether their ultimate resolution was the one they sought or not. The Vortex is not a friendly place; it's not a pleasant experience.

First of all, exhaust all possible means of resolving any dispute you have with school personnel at the school level. That means, talk to the teacher, the department head, the assistant principal and the principal before anyone else. Talk to your child's case manager (if you have one, and you should), the social worker, the guidance counselor and anyone who has been especially helpful to you and your child and who understands your child well. In my son's case, this was the speech and language specialist, until she left for another school system last year, a move that from time to time still makes me consider picketing her house.

"One of the first things I try to tell parents is that you try to create the relationship with someone on the (Child Study) Team beforehand," that very specialist says now. "No matter what you're walking into, you know you have someone who will listen to you."

There's a reason why resolving disputes is best done at the school level – they're more likely to be resolved to the parents' satisfaction. That doesn't mean you'll get everything you want, but forcing a school or district to a hearing outside the district is expensive for the school (and may be for you as well). It is difficult and time consuming, and the outcome is entirely out of your hands.

In the district, you can compromise, you can propose alternative solutions and you can find someone else to talk to about the problem. Outside the district, your options are limited, and the outcome is decided by someone other than yourself. The decision is usually final, and usually binding. And I've heard of cases in which, even when the parents got the decision they wanted, they found it more difficult to get the district to implement the changes wholeheartedly after a contentious and expensive process.

Let's assume for the sake of argument that you've been through the process in the school and your district, gone as far as the superintendent of schools (or headmaster, in private schools) and the board of education in your town, and you've gotten nowhere. Not just that you haven't gotten everything you've requested for your child, but that the essential, bottom-line services or accommodations your child needs to get through a day of school and have a chance to succeed have been denied.

If that's the case, you need to consider further options. Get in touch with a parent advocate (as discussed in the previous chapter) or an attorney. In fact, an attorney isn't a bad idea in such a case, but be sure it's one with a background in special education law. Most criminal or family law attorneys do not have the background you need, and therefore will not be able to give you and your child the help you need. Don't enter The Vortex with a handicap if you don't have to.

Ira Fingles, the disabilities rights attorney in the firm of Hinkle and Fingles in New Jersey and Pennsylvania, says that "school districts try to paint this picture that there's a black-and-white rule in many cases when there isn't one. Parents are better off understanding the procedures to avoid this (oversimplication)."

The procedures involve a move from personal contact with the district to communication through the attorney, and the beginning of proceedings that will probably start with a mediation, at which the school district and the parents (or the parents' attorney or advocate) present their sides of the argument. Finally, an independent, often state-appointed mediator makes a ruling based on the arguments. The ruling is binding, but if the parents believe it is in error, the mediation is not the last step in the process.

Parents can file for a due process hearing in court, and in that case, an attorney is almost absolutely essential. In this case, the decision will be final (barring appeals to higher courts), and the law is the issue at hand. "It's best not to get to this step," Fingles says, and "the preparation that goes into it is the same procedure that would be used in avoiding such a hearing."

"The ways to be prepared for a mediation or due process are the same ways to avoid a due process," he says. "You have to start by having a written record. Of everything."

Every communication between parents and a school or school district should be made in writing, and that writing should be preserved. If you speak to a teacher or school personnel of any kind on the phone, write a letter that begins, "to reiterate our conversation of (the date of the conversation) ..." And if you email someone in the school district, do not delete that email, and also keep a hard copy of it in a file somewhere else in your home.

"Having that written record is crucial," Fingles says. "Sometimes, it absolutely gets personal. I've witnessed it hundreds of times. And it's really hard for parents to not respond in kind. So having a written record of what was said and what the topic really was will make a huge difference. You can't prove it if it's not in writing."

The process in The Vortex will vary from state to state, and some areas are seen as friendlier to autism spectrum parents than others. "Vermont and Wisconsin are held out as model states," Fingles says, although I've spoken with parents from both states who disagree with that categorization. "The law will depend so much on what happens on the state level. It's not the same everywhere you go."

Preparing for any kind of hearing, even one within your school district, involves getting together every piece of written correspondence between you and anyone from the district. It involves a knowledge of what your state (or country) law says is necessary for children with disabilities. It requires that you be able to present your child's case, the reasons why the accommodations you're requesting are necessary, and the results you expect (given recommendations from experts in the field) to come from your child having the accommodations – and from not having them.

Listen to the advice of the attorney or advocate with whom you're working. Even if the answers you get aren't the ones you want to hear, remember that this is the person you chose to help your child. If he or she is advocating a solution that isn't exactly what you've been requesting, maybe you need to change your expectations.

The Vortex can be a grueling and difficult process, and even parents who end up with a decision in their children's favor often say they'd prefer not to have had to go through it. "We ended up with the judge (in a due process hearing) giving us pretty much everything we asked for," one Indiana parent told me. "But by then, the situation with the school system had gotten so nasty and so personal, I didn't want to deal with them any more, and I got the feeling they'd continue to fight me on every service they were now required to give (her son). We ended up moving to another district."

Fingles says it's important to remember that "the folks on 'the other side' are not the enemy. They're representing a system. Parents hear (the district) is difficult, and they come in with both barrels blazing, and that doesn't help. Don't make it personal with the school district, because that never helps."

One mom who lives in Massachusetts says her mediation ended up going in the school system's favor, and she believes it could have been avoided if the communication between the parents and the school hadn't become personal. "I regret that we didn't get an advocate," she says now. "It might have come out the same way, but it wouldn't have gotten as mean as it did."

Getting caught in The Vortex is a necessary evil in some cases – there's no other way to proceed if you have reached an impasse with your child's school. But even going to court with a district can be less antagonistic if you keep personality out of the proceedings.

It's important to remember that the goal isn't to "beat" the school system. It's to make sure your child gets the best possible chance to get the same education as everyone else in his school. If you have to enter The Vortex to do that, so be it. But enter with your eyes open and be sure you know what to expect. Arm yourself well, and hope you can keep those weapons in the holster.

Chapter Thirteen

YES, IT IS ALL ABOUT MONEY — OR NOT

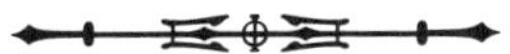

In the course of doing the research for this book, I was told countless times by parents that no matter what the terms of the disagreement with the school district were, "it's all about the money."

Yet, every single teacher, administrator, school psychologist, expert and state, city or federal official I spoke to, with no exceptions, said, "it's not all about money."

Well, the truth is, it's all about money. And, it's not.

School systems, especially those funded publicly, have to worry about their budgets. There's no questioning that. But most of them are mandated to provide the necessary services and accommodations to children who have any sort of a disability that could interfere with their ability to receive an education that is comparable to that of other children in the same school. Funding can come from state or federal government grants, from taxes or direct contributions from various governments, but it is available, one way or another. The way the system is set up, no public school is able to refuse services to a child who needs them because of budgetary constrictions.

"Truthfully, I don't believe (money) is the issue," says Ellyn Atherton, director of human resources for the Springfield, New Jersey, school system (and former speech and language specialist and director of educational services elsewhere). "If I went to my director, or to the superintendent and said, 'I truly believe that this is the best thing for this kid,' I think they're not going to say to me, 'how are we going to pay for it?'"

Some parents will disagree. One Pennsylvania mom told me in no uncertain terms that "the reason (my son) isn't getting the services he needs is that the school system doesn't have the money; I know it because that's what they told me." Her son, she believes, needs the attention of a one-on-one aide, and the school system in her district is not budgeted for another paraprofessional, she says a school employee has told her off the record.

And it's not limited to the United States. One mom in London says that she feels "it would be to (my son's) advantage to get a statement (of diagnosis, or a classification). At the end of the day, in my opinion, what it really means is an obligation for the Education Authority (the U.K. equivalent of the school district) to provide more staff and resources. It's all down to money, and I'm sure it's not too dissimilar in the States." No, it's really not.

Other parents around the country and in Canada have told me that "extra" services like ABA, "brushing," physical therapy and in some cases speech and language or occupational therapy have been deemed "too expensive" by their public school systems. The parents were advised either to pay for the services themselves, find a "charity organization" that would foot the bill, or have their children do without the services the parents, and not the school, considered necessary.

Money may be the root of all evil, but it pays for virtually every therapy and accommodation made for children on the autism spectrum in school, from special education classrooms, resource rooms, to services made available to children in "mainstream" classrooms. Like it or not, money in school budgets will make a difference to your child's success or lack of it in school, and knowing that at the outset should help you prepare for the discussions to come.

However, money doesn't have to come between your child and the services she requires. In fact, most public school systems are required by law to provide adequate services to all students who need them, no matter what the budget may say.

Some frequent complaints by some school systems – that hiring a full-time employee or providing a ground-breaking therapy for one child will create a prohibitive cost that will diminish the level of services for all the children in the district, or that "if we give it to you, we have to give it to everyone" – are easy to counter in most cases. First of all, if a service is required by everyone, it should and must be given to everyone under most states' laws. And if the district truly finds it prohibitively expensive to provide a service to one child only, it has an option: It can pay for that child to attend another school where the service is provided. Granted, some parents might not be interested in having their children attend a school for "special needs children," or might prefer that the child receive the services in-district, but the cost of sending a child to private school would, in most cases, be higher than that of the service itself, so it can become a moot point, and the child gets the service.

Even that idea is more adversarial than most parent-school relationships need to be. Atherton insists that schools in general are not more concerned with cost than they are with the children they serve. "In the back of your head, (money) is always an issue, but for most staff, it's asking for something they truly believe is necessary," she says. "The professionals I know are always more concerned with that."

However, sometimes money is an issue for parents, regardless of what the school system is or is not willing to offer in services and accommodations. For parents who opt for private school, especially, having a child on the spectrum can become a financial issue. And even for those whose children remain in public schools, the added responsibility of a child who has extra needs can manifest itself in issues of dollars and cents.

"I had to quit my job to help take care of my son," says one North Carolina parent. "We only have one income now, and we had just bought a house (when my son was diagnosed). Because of his difficulties in transitioning, he needs me to be there more than most kids do."

After an especially traumatic episode in school, in which her son was kept in "what they called a time-out room, but was really a closet," her son sometimes refuses to go to school at all. "Sometimes when we pull into the parking lot, he starts to scream, and I just pull out again," she says. "I couldn't do that if I was working full-time."

When money becomes an issue for a family with a child on the spectrum, like most problems, it is amplified. "I can't tell you what the divorce rate is (among parents with children on the spectrum)," says one support group president who asked not to be named, "but it's higher than the national average, I'm sure. I've heard an awful lot of stories. Sometimes it's denial on the part of one parent or the other, but a lot of the time, it's about money."

Financial help is sometimes available to parents on the spectrum, if in no other way than through before- and after-school help for when both parents have to work. Programs that care for children with early morning drop-off and late afternoon pick-up are available in most districts, and with a properly written IEP, such placement may be included in a child's program. And they can include the same accommodations and services that are given the child during the school day, to make it easier for the child and others in his class.

"We had to argue with the school over the after-school program," one Ohio mother told me. "They thought (my son) would be impossible to handle, because he gets more agitated as the school day goes on. But once they started preparing him properly, he realized he'd have help doing his homework, which was always a huge issue when he came home. Now, he goes happily."

The type of services and programs available to your child on the autism spectrum will to a great extent depend on the district in which you live. Financial considerations are a huge factor: A district with more money might be able to pay for more services for spectrum children. But in some cases, they may not. Some districts, with an eye toward keeping standardized test scores high, might prefer to send some children on the spectrum out of district and pay for services elsewhere. So it's no guarantee that a public school in an affluent district will be more amenable to paying for services or keeping children included than a school with a lower budget.

When trying to find the right school for a child, it's much more important to determine the district's philosophy of inclusion and services than it is to count the average annual income of the area. Teachers and administrators who understand the disorders, the behaviors and the effect they will have on children and schools – and who are more willing to be creative, thoughtful and understanding in their dealings with spectrum children and their parents – are much more effective with a child on the spectrum, no matter what the district's budget is.

"Our school doesn't have a lot of money," said one New Jersey father. "They don't have computers in every classroom, and as far as I know, they don't spend as much on each student as (a town nearby). But when we went in to talk to the principal the first day after our son was diagnosed, we knew she understood what the problem was, and she wanted to help (our son). And we have never had a problem with the school. I don't think the money has ever mattered. When he needed a full-time aide, the aide was there. When he needed OT, they had somebody to do that. We never had to figure out a way to pay for something. Money's never been an issue."

Some parents will read that paragraph and roll their eyes: It seems to come from another, simpler world where school systems don't ever turn down a request for special services for a child with an autism spectrum disorder. But it is true, and my own experience has been similar. Our son has been denied exactly one request in our 11 (so far) years of association with the local school system, and in retrospect, I understand why it was denied, even if it did make my life a little more difficult financially at the time. It was a financial issue, after all, and the school did offer a compromise measure that my wife and I felt was not the best thing for our son, so we refused it.

Aside from that incident, the local district has actually suggested services for our son. It has offered things that we didn't request. It has granted a full-time aide for the past seven years, and counting. Our son has had occupational therapy, social skills training, speech and language training and accommodations in some of his classes, some of the subtler ones like extra time on tests or the ability to take notes on a laptop computer lasting into his high school career. The issue of money has never been raised, aside from that one time, and even then, it wasn't the main source of disagreement, merely one aspect.

It can be done. The key, as with almost all other issues, is to find the school or the district that best understands your child's needs and will work to meet them. That's hard and sometimes requires extraordinary effort or lifestyle changes (I've known families who moved more than once to find a better school system). But when it's successful, it is the best possible situation for the child.

And that's what we're all after, isn't it?

Chapter Fourteen

TRY TO SEE THE OTHER SIDE

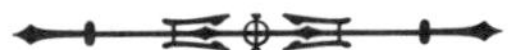

It's never easy. When someone seems to stand between you and what your child needs to succeed at school, you don't want to see that person's side of the argument. You have no inclination to understand his or her pressures, the things that go into his or her decision-making process, or the factors that make him or her feel that a way other than yours is best. Instead, you want that person to listen to you, to be persuaded, to comprehend that what you want is really what's best for your child.

The weird part is that's what that person is thinking, too.

In doing the research for this book, I have spoken to teachers, professionals who consult with school systems, principals, administrators and staff experts (psychologists, social workers, learning consultants, speech and language experts, and so on) who make decisions on a regular basis involving students on the autism spectrum, their parents, and the programs necessary to support those students in the school environment. Some were undereducated on the subject of autism and the latest techniques to help. Some felt hamstrung by budgetary matters or regulations. Some were convinced that they were dealing with some parents – not all parents – who were more concerned about winning the battle than helping the child.

But not one of the school personnel members I spoke to was an evil person.

It can sometimes seem that schools are going out of their way to be adversarial, that they begin the day wondering if there is a new way they can keep parents from securing services or accommodations. When you're in the heat of an argument, it's hard not to see as evil teachers who won't seat a tall student with Asperger Syndrome at the front of the room because that's where he will best be able to concentrate. It's hard not to believe that a principal who doesn't understand that a child with autism might be frightened by a fire drill and be unable to function for the rest of the day is being an autocrat. It's difficult to understand how a school psychologist can see a child who won't make eye contact, plays in isolation and is losing language by the day, yet won't cncur with a diagnosis of autism.

And still, these are not evil people. These are not people who want your child to fail at school, even if they believe your child would do better at another school. They do not really spend long meetings trying to find new ways to make your life miserable.

Not everyone is a sympathetic or empathetic person. Not all of them know exactly what autism is about, or why a child who seems to be obstinate really isn't trying to show them up in class. There are some, surely, who are not the best at what they do and consider the disruption of a student on the autism spectrum to be outside the normal limits, and unacceptable for the teacher and the rest of the class. Certainly, some believe we are coddling our children, putting "fancy labels" on behavior problems and not exercising a proper amount of discipline.

I don't by any measure discount the fact that some people who work in schools don't know enough about our children and don't care to know enough about our children. But the fact is, when you're trying to help your child through a school system, it is always helpful to see things through the eyes of the people with whom you are negotiating. What are their concerns? Why do they have objections to what you're proposing? How would their concerns be eased, and where do your interests coincide?

If you can answer those questions successfully before you go to, let's say, an IEP meeting, you are halfway to succeeding at what you're trying to do. Because persuasion is successful based on the degree to which you can convince the person who stands in your child's way that:

1. What you are proposing will help your child;
2. Helping your child will make it easier to help other children in class;
3. Helping other children in class will make everyone's job easier;
4. Your child will not be the last one to come through this school system with autism.

Negotiation – and quite often, asking for a particular service, therapy or accommodation will involve negotiation – is all about making the other person see the benefit to him in what you want. It's better yet if you can convince that person that the whole thing was his idea in the first place – more on that later. To begin with, it is important to view the situation through the school system's "eyes" and see where the difficulties lie, why people who work for the district might feel the way they do, and what can be done to convince them that your way will, in time, alleviate the problems they see, rather than creating more problems, which is their concern.

"When you show the principal, for example, that you understand your child might have a meltdown, you're exhibiting the ability to see their point of view," says a parent advocate from Missouri. "What you have to be able to show them is that with the proper safeguards and accommodations in place, your child will be less likely to have that meltdown, and emphasize that it's important because then every child in the room won't have to go through that meltdown, and neither will the teacher. That's what they're concerned about."

Emotionally, it can be difficult to step into the school official's shoes. Parents who have been through tough battles with their districts are already a little wary, and can be less than open to the idea that the school ever wants to do something beneficial for their children, or that any idea a teacher or professional who works for that district proposes might be good.

But, strictly from a strategic viewpoint, there are few things as effective as putting yourself in the "opponent's" position for a few minutes. First, it will help to anticipate arguments that might come up when you're trying to achieve something at a meeting. If you understand why an administrator isn't willing to provide advanced behavior analysis, you might be able to have a counterargument ready that will help persuade.

Beyond that, understanding the position of school personnel can help you to see if their resistance to some of your proposals might be reasonable. And even if they're not, you can see why the people who work for your district want something other than what you're requesting. You can empathize with them and see how the problems they see can be solved while still obtaining the necessary services.

For example, your child has Asperger Syndrome, and the sound of scratching on the holographic covers of the agenda notebooks your school hands out is extremely upsetting to him, causing him to put his hands over his ears and possibly have meltdowns in the classroom. You are calling the school principal to ask for an accommodation.

If you go in demanding that all the agenda books with the offending covers be turned in and replaced with books that don't have scratchy front panels, it would seem like an equitable solution to the problem. From your child's point of view.

However, the principal will note that the board of education in town has purchased 10,000 such agenda books, and they have been paid for. In addition, the books have already been distributed, and in use for days, weeks or months before your call. It's possible these are the same books that have been used in the system for years before your child started going to school here. For these reasons, the principal might not be able to understand how devastating a problem this can be for a young boy with AS.

In addition, even if the principal is sympathetic, she might not see a practical way to alleviate the problem. Recalling every agenda book in the district would seem an extreme reaction to one student's problem, and the financial consequences would certainly be questioned, not only by the board of education and the superintendent of schools, but by district residents as well. The principal has to answer to all these entities when making a policy decision, and while she might feel very strongly about helping your child through a day without the distraction, she might not be able to justify it to those above her in the district.

By seeing things from the other point of view, you can be ready with a solution that will satisfy all the parties involved: Either you can offer to supply, at your own expense, new agenda books for everyone in your child's classroom (assuming he is in a lower grade, where most subjects are taught in one classroom by one teacher), or you can supply everyone in your child's class with non-scratchy book covers to put over the agendas.

Because you are not demanding a solution that the principal would be unable to justify, you have a much better chance of acceptance. You can do something quickly and easily, without the protracted arguments, meetings, proposals and counterproposals that can ensue when each party is interested only in one solution, and neither party is willing to compromise at all.

Empathy, the ability to see things through another person's eyes, is a quality that we are sometimes told is difficult for children with autism spectrum disorders. If we as parents can exercise empathy to the degree that we can see things through the eyes of those who work in our school district, we will have a far better chance to help our children through the parts of the school day that they find more difficult than most.

"A lot of parents look at the (Child Study) Team as people they're going against," says one New Jersey mom. "I see them all as part of the team that's helping my child. Every time I go to an IEP meeting, I bring coffee." But her commitment and her ability to see the "other side" goes beyond that.

Her high-school-age son had been going to classes at a local college at night. He'd been having difficulty in high school because of some social aspects of the day, but in the college classes, her son thrived.

"I went to the district and said, 'I understand there have been problems, and here's a solution,'" she says. "They're treating (the college program) as an out-of-district placement. He goes to classes there, and (the school) pays the entire college tuition and all his supplies. I quoted a few sections of IDEA and the Free Appropriate Public Education (FAPE) sections, and within an hour after the meeting, they called to say, 'we're covering the books, too.' They're going to bus him to and from the college, and he's flourishing there. (The school personnel) think they might want to do this with some other kids in the district."

It can help to see things through another person's eyes, and it can be a good life lesson for our children, as well as for us.

Chapter Fifteen

REPORT CARDS

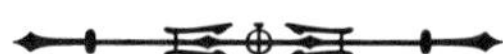

Having been through grade school (and, for many of us, high school, college and who knows what else), we understand the relative importance of grades. We know that our education is measured by the letter marks we get on quizzes, tests and final exams, and when we were younger, we probably spent at least some time sweating out the moment when one parent, guardian or other authority figure would read the latest of our report cards.

For many parents with children on the autism spectrum, this is a memory that is very difficult to share with our children. For people with Asperger Syndrome, like my son, there are two categories of subjects on this planet: What We're Interested In Beyond All Reason, and Who Cares? This can lead to a certain amount of confusion and difficulty when we're trying to motivate our children to do well in school. They wonder what will happen to them if they don't do well, and when we tell them that we'll still love them and they'll still live here and do all the things they do now, worrying about such obviously insignificant matters seems, well, insignificant.

A few years ago, when my son was in fifth grade, he came home with a report card that wasn't up to his usual "high-B" standards. Because I work at home, I'm the first one to see the report card. When I looked at his grade in English, a subject in which he'd always excelled, and told him I was disappointed with it, Josh seemed truly puzzled by my reaction.

"I got a C," he said. "That's average."

So, what was my problem? He was an average kid, in an average home, why not get average grades? And why should he care if his grade had actually dropped significantly from one marking period to the next? It was just a letter on a piece of paper. What difference could it make?

It's hard to impress upon a child with autism or a related disorder that grades can matter. Particularly for those who intend to go to college, grades in high school can make a huge difference in acceptance to the institution of their choice, and throughout a school career, the grades a student gets will help to determine which classes she will be able to attend in the following school term.

Do our kids care? Quite often, not really.

Sweating out the report card, then, never leaves us as parents with children on the spectrum. We worried about them when we were in school, and we worry about them now – although from a different perspective.

Luckily, our children often start out with no stress whatsoever about their report cards. The trick is to maintain that lack of tension while impressing upon the child that these things do matter, and that he must care about doing well on tests, projects and papers assigned in school.

It's a fine line to walk – if we make report cards sound too important, our children will (eventually) pick up on this, worry about pleasing us, and end up far more stressed out about their grades than they have to be in order to do well. If we de-emphasize the importance of good grades, or ignore them completely, on the other hand, our children will undoubtedly ignore the subject entirely, study hard on those subjects they find fascinating, and treat the others as nothing but annoyances and wastes of perfectly good school time.

The older my son gets, and the closer he gets toward applying to college, the more serious his concern about grades becomes. He started out with no concern at all, and, unfortunately, in our attempts to impress upon him that this issue did matter, my wife and I might have laid on the responsibility a little too thick. As I write this, he is going through his first round of final exams in high school, and Josh has been a little more stressed out than he needs to be for the past few weeks. Perhaps we did our job too well.

He knows that college is important, and he has a genuine desire to do well and to get to a school that will teach him about the subjects he finds fascinating, most of which have to do with video games and movies. But he also knows that in order to be accepted to good colleges, he will have to have a grade point average in high school that will attract attention, good scores on his SATs and some level of social and community activity. Applying to college is more competitive and in some ways more difficult than it was when I applied in 1975.

The problem is, Josh knows this all too well. He feels that if he doesn't do well on his freshman-year final exams, he will be hurting his chances of getting to a good college, and despite our assurances that he'll do fine, and that there are plenty of colleges and he'll find one, he has been tense and irritable for the weeks leading up to his exams. Had this been two years ago, he would have been absolutely unconcerned, and probably would do very well on his exams, since he wouldn't be the least bit worried about them; besides, the work was less difficult two years ago than it is at his current level.

Josh has always believed that he should concentrate on the things that come most easily to him, especially since they are the ones he finds the most interesting (not surprisingly). So we had to take steps to impress upon him the importance of trying and studying, and not just doing the least he could do to get by in classes in which he was not naturally engaged.

Toward that end, we began in his early grades offering rewards for doing some work on his projects or homework, or for studying before a test (although in very early grades, little studying was required; we just wanted him to get into the habit). Because my son has never in his life, even at age 3, responded to such things as gold stars or stickers, they had to be tangible rewards like points toward a game he wanted or – yes, I know I'm a bad parent – a Dunkin Donut for studying or working on a project.

Homework, early on, was a struggle, and one that I'll discuss in more detail in a later chapter. But suffice it to say that a very strict routine had to be established to make things work right, and once it was implemented, it was extremely effective, and remains in place to this day. If you're really interested, skip ahead to Chapter Twenty-Five.

Studying, however, was and always has been another story.

Like many children (my definition of kids with Asperger Syndrome is that they're just like everyone else, only more), children with spectrum disorders are not given to studying simply for the thrill of learning new information. They are, in fact, struck with a distinct disdain for studying, seeing it as a waste of time and effort when such important things as television, video games and sleeping could be part of the schedule.

In this connection, it's a sad fact that study skills are, generally speaking, not taught as part of the average school curriculum. Kids don't really understand the concept of repetition in studying, the fact that it will take longer than 10 minutes to memorize or understand a new concept. Having not been taught the skill, they understandably find it hard to put into action.

Motivation, then, becomes important. For most children, the immediate consequence of a bad grade, or a special small reward for getting a good one, is enough to drive the concept of studying into the "relevant" file. For children with spectrum disorders, however, "relevant" is harder to achieve. They need structure in their lives, so studying, even if a test is not imminent, must become part of that routine, something that is not questioned or ignored because of convenience: Even if the child is going out to a family dinner that night, studying has to be worked into the daily schedule somehow.

That's important: Studying subjects, even when homework is not assigned for the day, should be part of a daily schedule. Saving it for only those times when a test is imminent increases the stress level for the student and, worse for children with an autism spectrum disorder, disrupts the routine, forcing not only an activity that might not be the child's favorite thing to do, but also a change in the daily order of things they find comforting and necessary.

If your child has not yet started school, or is young enough that a daily routine for school has not been set in stone, please take that as a warning: Take steps as early as possible to establish studying, even if it's just called "practice" at the beginning, as a vital part of a daily script for your child's school life. Make sure it's not questionable or variable: At a certain time each day, a time of day when your child is likely to be open to such things, make sure some "practice" is done. It doesn't have to be a lot, and it doesn't have to be complicated. It just has to be.

If your child has been going to school for a while without that mandatory time spent each day, introduce it as soon as you can. Do it when there is no big test on its way, when there's no stressful situation imminent, just when your child is well prepared for a new part of the daily routine. Start by talking about it for a couple of weeks before you start, and participate with the student if you find that helpful – use flash cards, quizzes, rewards, whatever it takes to make the idea acceptable, but do it right away.

Also, establish the idea that grades matter. Not in a threatening or worrisome way, but by pointing to a future that includes the things your child wants, whatever they might be. Grades are not a way to compare your child to other children ("look, Karen got a B and you only got a C") but a way to show the child how well he is doing in school, by comparison only to himself ("you got a D the last time, and now it's up to a C!"). Make sure your child understands that you think the report card is important; eventually, he will probably come around to understand that point of view. Probably.

Even if he doesn't, knowing that you do might be enough. Grading is a difficult concept for any child to accept, and our children are less inclined to find it exciting and fun to be compared to their neurotypical peers. But making the point that you feel it's important to try hard and accomplish what the student can will provide some incentive, especially in younger children, and once the pattern is established, a child on the spectrum will probably not deviate from it without some serious reason to do so.

It's always easier to get a child on the spectrum to try harder when the subject is one that interests her, or when the method of teaching is one the child considers enjoyable. You know your child better than anyone; you can probably find ways to make the experience a smoother and more pleasant one for everybody.

That doesn't mean it's going to be easy. You know perfectly well that when you have a child with a disorder on the autism spectrum, nothing is going to be easy. But studying and working for better grades doesn't have to be an unpleasant, difficult experience. As with anything else we do, it's better when serious thought is given ahead of time, and the child is well prepared in advance for any methods you might want to employ.

Hang in there. Eventually, they graduate.

Chapter Sixteen

TEASING

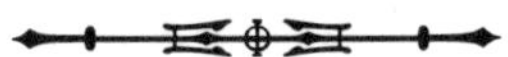

In 1998, when my son was 9 years old, I wrote an article about Asperger Syndrome (and, by extension, my son) for *USA Weekend*, the Sunday newspaper supplement for Gannett newspapers. Before I agreed to write the article, I asked Josh if he was uncomfortable with my mentioning his spectrum disorder to 34 million people on a Sunday morning.

He thought about the implications for a while, then came back to talk about it and had only one question: "Will the bullies see it?"

Teasing is a fact of life on the autism spectrum. Because our children don't exhibit "visible" signs of a physical disorder, they are not seen in the same light as those in wheelchairs or holding white canes. That's fine, since the spectrum does not mean the same kind of physical barriers or obstacles as more "visible" disorders.

However, because other children can't see autism or Asperger Syndrome, they see only the behaviors that result from the disorder: self-stimming behaviors, "different" reactions to stimuli, uncomfortable moments and sometimes awkward conversations. Our children are considered "the weird kids" in class.

When I was in grade school, there was a boy in my class named, let's say, Edgar. He didn't really know how to talk to the rest of us, but never stopped talking. He had unconventional ideas about science, like the notion that aliens from other planets were among us on earth. He was gawky and physically clumsy. In retrospect, it seems to me that he probably had an autism spectrum disorder.

We teased him mercilessly, and I'm ashamed to say, I did not stick up for him in the least.

Now, raising an "Edgar" of my own for the past 15 years, I have become more sensitive to the sadness and humiliation that goes with the teasing. All of us feel put upon when we're in school at one time or another, and children on the spectrum are, again, just like everyone else – only more.

It can become far more than a simple case or two of one child poking fun at another. Teasing is a legitimate problem for children on the spectrum, one that demands action before it escalates into something much more serious.

When children see that a child acts differently, they often react with taunts and teasing. In the middle grades, this can become especially vicious. The child with the spectrum disorder is often caught between two bad alternatives: either show weakness and allow the teasing to escalate, or react badly and face disciplinary action or, in some cases, violence and injury to the child or a classmate.

Parental reaction (and, in some cases, action) has often taken the form of defense, trying to help the child with a spectrum disorder out of trouble after an incident has occurred at school. School reaction is just as often reactive, as teachers and administrators generally don't act on a problem with behavior until it has crossed the line from potential situation to real situation.

Some parents have tried to head problems off before they begin with what one friend of mine calls a "dog-and-pony show," a program aimed at younger children that explains (sometimes with a psychologist or other outside expert coming to school to speak) the disorder and why a particular child will act differently in many situations than most. Video programs like *Intricate Minds: Understanding Classmates With Asperger Syndrome* (www.coultervideo.com), being distributed through some support group organizations (www.aspennj.org), go further, explaining the disorder but also illustrating with comments from children who have an autism spectrum disorder, to put a face on the unfamiliar words the school audience is hearing for the first time, in many cases.

"We make every teacher (my son will have) watch a three-hour Tony Attwood video," says a Virginia-based mother. "The majority of his teachers have been astoundingly wonderful after that, but we didn't want to leave it up to the school to do the training."

Of course, such efforts can backfire, giving classmates more ammunition in the teasing wars. But for the most part, explaining to children why a classmate acts in an unusual fashion and suggesting ways to help that child get through what can be a difficult school day is an effective way of cutting back on teasing and sometimes forging friendships among children with spectrum disorders and their peers.

Another plan can take on the look of something like Peer Buddies, which Sharie Ostrowski, a Washington state mom, introduced to me. Sharie learned about Peer Buddies from another area parent with a child on the autism spectrum, and each of them is working to spread the word about the program throughout the autism community.

Peer Buddies is a cooperative effort by the teachers and students in the classroom of a child with a spectrum disorder. It begins with a carefully planned explanation to the class by a teacher, the school nurse or another school staff member, outlining the program and the background of autism and related disorders. It is often started in early grades, when children are more open to suggestions and less concerned with what is and is not "cool." Younger children seem to be more accepting to differences among peers when they are well explained.

"They are so kind to my son once they understand why he acts a little bit odd sometimes," Sharie says. "Sometimes his behavior comes off as being rude when he just doesn't know how to communicate properly. They accept that, and they don't get mad or take offense. There have not been any cases of bullying to my knowledge when the (Peer Buddies) program is going on."

Once the class has been through the orientation program, each child is eligible to sign up and indicate interest in becoming a Peer Buddy for the child in class with a spectrum disorder. The classroom teacher, aide or other adult running the program sifts through the names of children who volunteer and choose the ones they think will be best suited to the program.

"In (my son's) first grade (class), all the children were interested, and they all signed up," Sharie recalls. "They were so enthusiastic. But this year, the teacher decided it was a little difficult having all the kids be Peer Buddies, so she was careful to stress that this was a huge responsibility, and they got a more selective group."

Once a child has been selected, a letter with a permission slip is sent to his or her parents, and if the parents agree, the child is then given some orientation to the Peer Buddy program. "They get out a white board and they list what (my son's) strengths are and what his difficulties are," Sharie says. "How they can help him, and the kids are expected to spend time with him during unstructured time at school, recess and lunch, basically."

She says the program has been an enormous help for her son and others she has seen in the Peer Buddy program. "They sit with him at an assembly, or they help him to get redirected. After the orientation, when they're doing the white board and all that, we pull (my son) out."

With each year in school, Sharie tries to make the information she gives the class a little more age appropriate, and while her son is still in the early grades at school, she has seen a difference in the way his peers treat him.

"At one assembly, they were having a concert, and (my son) was stretching his arms out and acting in a way that's inappropriate for a concert," she recalls. (The Peer Buddy) "just reached over and put his arms back down at his sides, just to remind him."

Peer Buddies is just one of a large number of programs designed to help neurotypical children understand the autism spectrum a little better by interacting with and supporting children with special needs.

But it's not always that easy to dissuade children from teasing a classmate with a spectrum disorder, especially as they get older. "The middle school years are the worst," one teacher in New York state told me. "It's hard for any kid to get through those years, with all the exclusion that goes on. But for a kid with a difference, especially one you can't look at, one they haven't been told all their lives that you can't make fun of, it's harder. These kids are fair game."

That kind of situation can lead to extremely difficult moments, and as the children get older, bigger and more adolescent, teasing goes beyond words, and can sometimes end up becoming physical. For teenagers on the autism spectrum, whose impulse control isn't always on par with those of their neurotypical peers, school policies of zero tolerance can be dangerous. This is where teasing gets serious.

Schools can only do so much, but in many cases, they're not doing anything, and that gets some parents angry. "My son got into a fight with another boy because the other boy was baiting him," one New Jersey mother told me. "But the other kid knew how to do it only when the teachers weren't looking, and (my son) wasn't that subtle. Guess who got suspended?"

My son, who went through his serious moments of being teased in early grades, still has difficulty reacting to teasing, even when it might be good natured. Teenagers tend to tease each other, but they don't all react by threatening to throw chairs. This can lead to difficulties in school.

Because of zero-tolerance policies, and the intention of the school district to alert local authorities any time such policies are violated, we have asked for and gotten an assurance – written into my son's IEP – that we will be informed before any other action is taken involving our son and a reaction to pressure from classmates. I hasten to note that we've never had to use that provision, and fully expect that we never will; our son has never threatened another child, although he still does seem to find the least socially acceptable way to react to most stressful situations. His idea of showing frustration is to pick up a large chair and throw it to the floor. It attracts attention, but hasn't hurt anyone so far.

In 2001, a week after the attacks on the World Trade Center less than an hour from where we live, my son, in a fit of frustration, chose to tell one of his teachers that he would like to burn down the school. Tensions were understandably high at that moment, but luckily the teacher knew Josh pretty well, understood that he meant that only figuratively, and did not pursue it any further. Had it been someone who didn't understand him, he could have been prosecuted for making terroristic threats, and especially in those difficult days, it was not hard to imagine such a step being taken. Later that week, when a student actually did set a fire in one of the bathrooms, we were relieved that our son was with three teachers at the time the alarm bells rang, and therefore did not fall under any suspicion. Forget that he probably would have had a hard time lighting a match in those days. His fine-motor skills were still a little underdeveloped.

Teasing is a fact of life in school – it will never go away. We can help prepare our children for it with books and conversations. We can prepare their peers that our children might react differently than they would to certain situations, that they might seem "weird" or say things that seem rude. We can give the class scientific explanations of autism and related disorders and ask them to understand and act appropriately. Still, teasing will happen. It happens to neurotypical children, and it will happen – in all likelihood, more often – to ours.

Working with schools and school personnel, we can plan in advance for the best possible reaction to the inevitable teasing. We can minimize the hurt our children will feel, and we can maximize the chances (for example, through Social Stories™ and social skills training) that they will react in as appropriate a manner as possible.

It's like most other things involving autism and related disorders: Prior planning can help, but not cure. But in this case, the planning involves not only the child with the disorder, but all his classmates and peers as well. It won't be easy, but since when did we expect anything to be easy?

Chapter Seventeen

THE IEP MEETING

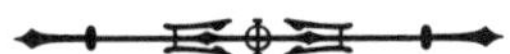

Cross a parent-teacher conference with a tax audit and throw in a trip to the dentist, and you'll have a vague approximation of what an IEP meeting sometimes feels like.

What most of us refer to as "The IEP meeting" is really an annual (or in some states, less often) review of a document (the Individualized Education Program) in place already. The fact is that under most states' laws, parents can request – and must be allowed – an IEP meeting whenever they believe it is necessary.

For many parents with children on the autism spectrum, the IEP meeting is like a visit to the principal's office, which it is, literally, in many cases. We feel like we're being called in to discuss our failings, to review the ways our children have misbehaved and underachieved during the school year, and the ways in which we as parents should have done something to prevent that.

To be fair, there are school systems in which the administrative staff and others reinforce that feeling. More than one parent told me of IEP meetings at which they were told that their children did not have a disorder related to autism, but were merely "behavior problems" resulting, in all likelihood, from parents who were too lenient and "didn't understand how to discipline children."

Well, that's wrong. Most of us are not coddling our children; if anything, we are asking them to do more than their neurotypical peers, because we are requiring them to get an education at the same time they are learning the behaviors and social skills that most other children acquire naturally.

But one area in which we parents do sometimes err is in allowing such school employees to have that much influence over us to begin with. We can't allow ourselves to enter an IEP meeting with the feeling that we're being reviewed, or even that the people with whom we're meeting have the authority to review us. We are supposed to be part of a team – a team that includes parents, teachers, administrators, professionals and, if necessary, school board members and local officials. But we are no less a part of the team than any other member, and we are reviewing how well the IEP is working, not how well we are doing as parents. If something's wrong, it is wrong with the document, and the meeting is meant to act as a review to change or strengthen any area that isn't working well enough at the present time.

That said, I'm not reversing gears here and advocating a first-strike attitude with Guns A' Blazing at the first IEP meeting, or any other, when it's not necessary. The first alteration in attitude has to be our own; we can't expect that those with whom we're meeting will treat us as anything but underachievers if we ourselves believe we are just that. We need to prepare for an IEP meeting, to be ready with facts and figures, if necessary, and to enter the room knowing that we are probably the best-informed people in the room on the subject of our children. We might be the best informed on autism and related disorders, but we can't be sure that's the case. We can be sure we're ready, if we've prepared properly.

An IEP meeting usually includes members of the Child Study Team – the school's psychologist, the social worker, a special education teacher, a general education teacher, perhaps a learning consultant – as well as parents. In most cases, it does not include someone whose background is based entirely in autism and its related disorders. So we need to gather as much information as we can on the subject, particularly the disorder with which our children have been diagnosed, and have it ready when we enter the meeting. It will help to illustrate points, and may inform everyone in the room on therapies and strategies they might not have considered, but that have worked for other children under similar circumstances.

It also can be extremely helpful to talk to some members of the team before the meeting, to gauge the mood, see where there might be disagreements or changes that need to be made in the IEP, so you can be prepared with an opinion and data to back it up. The teacher or staff member who is most familiar with your child, and who has (hopefully) been the most helpful to date, is your best bet. Call a few weeks before the meeting is scheduled to take place, discuss the school year, and find out where your child's strengths and weaknesses have been determined. See if the evaluations you hear discussed match your own opinions. See if the issues you raise are the same as those being raised by the school, and if not, whether your concerns seem to be meeting with acceptance or resistance.

Start by reviewing the previous IEP, the one that is in place for your child before the upcoming meeting. Read through it, note where the solutions to problems have been implemented, and whether you think they've been successful or not. Consider other areas that have not been addressed, and decide whether you think they need mentioning at the upcoming meeting. If a therapy or accommodation has been written into the current IEP, but is not being put into effect immediately, find out why that has not happened – don't wait until the meeting to implement strategies that have already been agreed upon.

Sometimes when a child has made significant progress with a plan, an IEP can be adjusted to eliminate therapies (speech and language, occupational therapy) that might no longer be necessary. But before you enter the annual meeting, be sure that you are comfortable with stopping a given accommodation; that your child will do as well without it. As mentioned earlier, it's not impossible to get a therapy reinstated if the child proves to need it after you and the Child Study Team determine it is unnecessary, but it's not easy. Better to err on the side of caution and continue something longer than it appears to be necessary than end something that's working well before the child is ready.

If this is the first IEP meeting you'll be attending, your concerns will be somewhat different, but the goal will be the same. In this case, of course, you won't be able to refer to the previous IEP, since none exists. But you might be able to read books and articles on the subject or to get a copy of a blank IEP form from the school, so you can determine how you think it should be completed to best help your child. Familiarize yourself with the language and the areas an IEP covers and doesn't cover, and be ready to offer suggestions on all the sections, even if they don't directly apply to your child's disorder.

One mother in Toronto, Canada, told me she takes a preemptive measure every year before attending the IEP meeting for her daughter. "Every time an IEP is due, I write an entire one and submit it to (the school)," she says. "What I am giving them is so specific. I've found that it's best to let them think it's their idea."

A New York-based teacher says that she likes to meet with parents ahead of the meeting and determine where any areas of disagreement might be, and to determine what is best for the child. "Before I write an IEP for one of my students, I sit down with the parents," she explains. "It's a very collaborative effort with the parents."

Once the meeting begins, the discussion is usually pretty informal. Parents can add suggestions at any time, and don't have to wait until their "turn" comes around. You will be asked to sign a form at the beginning of the meeting to acknowledge that you were present. Signing that form does not indicate your agreement with the IEP being devised at the meeting. You'll have a chance to agree or disagree with the final document later.

The meeting will progress with the school representatives making their recommendations – and that's all they are, recommendations – and explaining why they think this is the best plan for your child. You can ask all the questions you like, disagree when you don't feel the plan will help, and offer your own suggestions for therapies, accommodations and any other plans that you think will help your child succeed in school. Remember, the goal is not to make it easier for your child than other children or to give your child an unfair advantage. The IEP exists to level the playing field and help overcome the obstacles that your child's autism spectrum disability may present, in order to give your child the same chance at a good education as every other child in the school.

Occasionally, a disagreement about a suggestion, either from you or from a member of the school's Child Study Team, may arise. This is where the "no guns" approach is best used: If you assume the school is trying to deprive your child of a necessary service before there is any evidence to that effect, you will spoil your child's chance at a workable IEP. You may also jeopardize your relationship with the school district, which could cause problems for years to come for your child, you, and every teacher or administrator in the system. In that order.

Try instead to hear the school representatives' point of view, determine why they feel this is the best thing, and consider it. If the idea still strikes you as detrimental to your child's education, say so, but don't make the argument personal. A clash of personalities is the thing that most often poisons the parent-school relationship. And it is not necessary.

Once the IEP has been written, based on the suggestions made at the meeting, it should meet your satisfaction as well as that of everyone else at the meeting. If you disagree with any part of the finished document, which you have every opportunity to read, you are not required to agree to it. In fact, you should definitely not agree to a plan that you feel won't help your child. Remember that it doesn't have to be the best possible plan in the world; it has to be adequate to meet your child's needs. Anything less is unacceptable.

Should you decide that the IEP as written is not workable, that your child will be at a disadvantage because of provisions written into or left out of the document, you need to understand the procedure to make the desired changes. Many parents believe that they have to sign the IEP itself for the document to go into effect; that is, they think that unless they physically write their names on the IEP statement, it isn't valid and won't be implemented. This is only true of the child's *first* IEP.

In most districts, parents are mailed or given a copy of the IEP after it is completed, and from the second IEP on, if they don't raise their concerns and announce in writing their dissatisfaction with the IEP within 15 days of receiving it, it will be implemented as written.

Should you fail to do that, that's not the biggest tragedy that ever happened, since you can call for a new IEP meeting at any time. However, if you disagree strongly with the written document, document your dissatisfaction in a letter to the principal, your child's case manager, every name listed on the IEP and the superintendent of schools, as well as your child's teacher. Do it before the 15-day period, and the IEP will automatically be reconsidered. And yes, you will be included in the re-evaluation process.

"When they pushed to pull (my son) out of the classroom, I learned the power of the IEP," says a Missouri mom whose son is in public school. "The withholding of your signature on that document causes all kinds of problems for (the school district). My question persistently was, 'I understand that's difficult, but how are you going to get it done?' I was nice but I was persistent. Somebody at the district level saw there was no (signed) IEP, and their butts were all in slings."

Maybe that's not the image you have in mind, but you should be clear on one thing: An IEP that doesn't help your child isn't acceptable, and you don't have to agree to it. Put your disagreement in writing, and press on from there.

An IEP meeting doesn't have to be something a parent dreads. With the right attitude and a little persistence, it's possible to enjoy the experience. Not incredibly likely, but possible.

Chapter Eighteen

THE INVISIBILITY FACTOR

"I kept getting these notes home," one New Jersey mother says of her son. "They'd say, he's biting, he's this, he's that. I went into the classroom, and they were strapping him into a Rifkin (restraint) chair. Once they pulled me off the ceiling, I went in and we had an IEP meeting. I told them that if I found them restraining him again, I would call DYFS (Department of Youth and Family Services)."

Her family went further than that – in fact, they moved twice before finding a district in which her child has been thriving. But the level of misunderstanding and misconception in some places, in some schools, in some people, is unsettling.

Some teachers just don't "get" autism and its related disorders. They don't understand that it's not simply a question of children who are obstinate and stubborn. They don't believe that we, as parents, are not being unreasonable and expecting unusually favorable treatment for our children. They think we really don't know how to "discipline" a child, that we're being lenient and passive, allowing our children to run our families and our lives because we've bought into some buck-passing "excuse" for their behavior.

It's the difference between what a child won't do and what a child can't do that is difficult for some people – even some good teachers and administrators – to comprehend.

Think about it: You've been a teacher for 10 years. Or 20. Or five. Nobody has ever mentioned the words "Asperger Syndrome" to you. You've heard of "autism," but that's something that belongs in the special ed department. What you see before you is a child who seems to be very intelligent, but who refuses to listen to your instructions, has a difficult time sitting in his seat for any length of time, makes indistinguishable noises that distract the other students and, when confronted about his behavior, tends to get extremely agitated and either blames you for the problem or becomes so angry that he is no longer reasonable.

It's understandable – although not excusable – that such a teacher might not be receptive to discussing autism or other spectrum disorders. But does that mean a teacher who sees such students as behavior problems, distractions and detriments to the class' education has a point?

Of course not.

With the amount of information available today, with the kind of programs in place and with the responsibility a good teacher should feel about educating all the students in the classroom, there is no excuse for not understanding or tolerating students with autism or related disorders. It is the educator's responsibility to stay current on such issues, to try to help every student in the class and to put in a special effort for students who need extra help. Some teachers are not good teachers, and a lack of talent is certainly a problem. But refusing to pay attention to students who need assistance or extra understanding is simply wrong, and should be the last thing a responsible school district or administrator wants to see under his or her watch.

With that said, there are still teachers in public and private schools who do not recognize or understand autism spectrum disorders and the behavior they sometimes cause. There are plenty of horror stories out there, and many of them involve teachers who put on blinders and the administrators who back them up.

Parents have told me about teachers who call to complain about their children's behavior. They've mentioned teachers who have told them directly that the children shouldn't be in a mainstream classroom, or that the children belong, but are deliberately trying to disrupt the class. One mother of a boy with Asperger Syndrome told me that a principal, when told that a teacher was refusing to allow a child in her classroom until he stopped rapping his knuckles rhythmically on the desk, shrugged his shoulders and responded, "well, it's her classroom."

It's often said that autism spectrum disorders are "invisible," that they are difficult to explain and to spot because the children don't look any different than others, and that their behavior, except in some cases, is not so extreme that it is considered anything other than odd or irritating by classmates and teachers.

The Invisibility Factor can play against parents whose children have disorders on the spectrum, because it makes the case for special accommodations, services or therapies more difficult to make. It makes explaining our children's "peculiarities" to teachers harder, particularly to teachers who are less than receptive to the explanations we offer. Those teachers, the ones who just don't "get it," are the ones who will say that the neurological condition we are describing can't be all that serious, because the child is capable of paying attention when interested, and can do the academic work handed to him when he understands the instructions.

In short, sometimes The Invisibility Factor is simply a refusal to see what's there, rather than an inability to see what's there. It's an important distinction, since a teacher (or principal, or social worker, etc.) who wants to help and wants to understand will be infinitely more receptive to explanation and information than one who doesn't.

Those teachers can be helped with the aid of teaching tools that spell out the needs of students with disorders on the spectrum. One of the best I've ever seen is one written by Susan

Moreno and Carol O'Neal of MAAP Services for Autism and Asperger Syndrome that, with gracious permission, I reprint below. I have distributed it to every teacher my son has had since I discovered it. I think it presents its information in the clearest, most understandable language I've seen. It is a very helpful piece of work. I wish I'd written it.

Tips For Teaching High-Functioning People With Autism

By Susan Moreno and Carol O'Neal

1. People with autism have **trouble with organizational skills,** regardless of their intelligence and/or age. Even a "straight A" student with autism who has a photographic memory can be incapable of remembering to bring a pencil to class or of remembering a deadline for an assignment. In such cases, aid should be provided in the least restrictive way possible. Strategies could include having the student put a picture of a pencil on the cover of his notebook or reminders at the end of the day of assignments to be completed at home. Always praise the student when he remembers something he has previously forgotten. Never denigrate or "harp" at him when he fails. A lecture on the subject will not only NOT help, it will often make the problem worse. He may begin to believe he can't remember to do or bring these things.

   These students seem to have either the neatest or the messiest desks or lockers in the school. The one with the neatest desk or locker is probably very insistent on sameness and will be very upset if someone disturbs the order he has created. The one with the messiest desk will need your help in frequent cleanups of the desk or locker so that he may find things. Simply remember that he is not making a conscious choice to be messy, he is most likely incapable of this organizational task without specific training. Train him in organizational skills using small, specific steps.

2. People with autism have **problems with abstract and conceptual thinking.** Some may eventually acquire a few abstract skills, but others never will. Avoid abstract ideas when possible. When abstract concepts must be used, use visual cues, such as gestures, or written words to augment the abstract idea.

3. **An increase in unusual or difficult behaviors probably indicates an increase in stress.** Sometimes stress is caused by feeling a loss of control. When this occurs, the "safe place" or "safe person" may come in handy, because many times the stress will only be alleviated when the student physically removes himself from the stressful event or situation. If this occurs, a program should be set up to assist the student in re-entering and/or staying in the stressful situation.

4. **Don't take misbehaviors personally.** The high-functioning person with autism is not a manipulative, scheming person who is trying to make life difficult. Usually misbehavior is the result of efforts to survive experiences which may be confusing, disorienting, or frightening. People with autism are, by virtue of their disorder, egocentric and have extreme difficulty reading the reactions of others. *They are incapable of being manipulative.*

5. Most high-functioning people with autism **use and interpret speech literally.** Until you know the capabilities of the individual, you should avoid:
   - Idioms (save your breath, jump the gun, second thoughts, etc.)
   - Double meanings (most jokes have double meanings)
   - Sarcasm, such as saying, "Great!" after he has just spilled a bottle of ketchup on the table
   - Nicknames
   - "Cute" names such as Pal, Buddy, Wise Guy, etc.

6. **Be as concrete as possible** in all your interactions with these students. Remember that facial expression and other social cues may not work. Avoid asking questions such as, "Why did you do that?" Instead, say, "I didn't like the way you slammed your book on the desk when I said it was time for gym. Please put your book down on the desk quietly and get up to leave for gym." In answering essay questions that require a synthesis of information, autistic individuals rarely know when they have said enough, or if they are properly addressing the core of the question.

7. If the student doesn't seem to be able to learn a task, **break it down into smaller steps** or present the task in several different ways (e.g., visually, verbally, physically).

8. **Avoid verbal overload.** Be clear. Use shorter sentences if you perceive that the student isn't fully understanding you. Although he probably has no hearing problem and may be paying attention, he may have a problem understanding your main point and identifying the important information.

9. **Prepare the student for all environmental and/or routine changes,** such as assembly, substitute teacher, rescheduling, etc. Use his written or verbal schedule to prepare him for change.

10. Behavior management works, but if incorrectly used, it can encourage robot-like behavior, provide only a short-term behavior change, or result in more aggression. **Use positive and chronologically age-appropriate behavior procedures.**

11. **Consistent treatment** and expectations from **everyone** is vital.

12. Be aware that normal **levels of auditory and visual input can be perceived by the student as too much or too little.** For example, the hum of fluorescent lighting is extremely distracting for some people with autism. Consider environmental changes such as removing some of the "visual clutter" from the room or seating changes if the student seems distracted or upset by his classroom environment.

13. If your high-functioning student with autism uses **repetitive verbal arguments** and/or repetitive verbal questions, try requesting that he write down the question or argumentative statement. Then write down your reply. As the writing continues, the person with autism usually begins to calm down and stop the repetitive activity. If that doesn't work, write down his repetitive verbal question or argument, and then ask him to formulate and write down a logical reply or a reply he thinks you would make. This distracts him

from the escalating verbal aspect of the argument or question and sometimes gives him a more socially acceptable way of expressing his frustration or anxiety. If the student does not read or write, try role playing the repetitive verbal question or argument, with you taking their part and them answering you.

Continually responding in a logical manner or arguing back seldom stops this behavior. The subject of their argument or question is not always the subject that has upset them. The argument or question more often communicates a feeling of loss of control or uncertainty about someone or something in the environment. Individuals with autism often have trouble "getting" your points. If the repetitive verbal argument or question persists, consider the possibility that he is very concerned about the topic and does not know how to rephrase the question or comment to get the information he needs.

14. Since these individuals experience various communication difficulties, **don't rely on the students with autism to relay important messages** to their parents about school events, assignments, school rules, etc., unless you try it on an experimental basis with follow-up, or unless you are already certain that the student has mastered this skill. Even sending home a note for his parent may not work. The student may not remember to deliver the note or may lose it before reaching home. Phone calls to the parent work best until this skill can be developed. Frequent and accurate communication between the teacher and parent (or primary care-giver) is very important.

15. If your class involves **pairing off** or choosing partners, either draw numbers or use some other arbitrary means of pairing. Or ask an especially kind student if he or she would agree to choose the individual with autism as a partner. This should be arranged before the pairing is done. The student with autism is most often the individual left with no partner. This is unfortunate since **these students could benefit most from having a partner.**

I've had teachers and school administrators ask me for copies of the above document (which can also be found at the web site of O.A.S.I.S. (Online Asperger Syndrome Information and Support), http://www.udel.edu/bkirby/asperger/moreno_tips_for_teaching.html.

For teachers and school personnel who are unwilling to see The Invisibility Factor for what it is, the answer is simple: You have to go over their heads. Writing letters (writing is always better than calling) to the next person up the ladder (department head, principal, assistant superintendent, superintendent, and so on) delineating exactly what the problem has been – without any personal comments about the staff member you're discussing – is the best way to draw attention to the difficulty, and start getting the help your child needs.

Sometimes it's best to have your child moved to another class, where the teacher is more sensitive to students with special needs. If the principal of the school agrees, that won't be a problem, but it could be difficult for your child, as any disruption in routine is always problematical.

But in any case, it's extremely important to keep the personality issues – no matter how hurtful things might have become – out of any correspondence you send to help your child. Keep everything on a professional level, discuss the difficulties your child has been having, and suggest exactly how you believe they can be eased. Set a specific timetable, ask for a response as soon as possible, and follow up with a telephone call two or three days later if you've had no response.

Some teachers don't get The Invisibility Factor. That doesn't mean your child has to become invisible. It means the teacher has to be educated, or be replaced.

Chapter Nineteen

WHEN SHOULD MY GUN BE BLAZING?

I've been emphasizing the importance of not entering a relationship with a school system with your Guns A' Blazing. You've read enough about how to hold your frustration in check, how to see the other side of every argument and how to maintain a calm and professional attitude when speaking with or writing to teachers, principals, administrators, superintendents, boards of education and school professionals.

However, aren't there times when you shouldn't simply turn the other cheek? Don't some people who work for schools cross the line and make things personal, and shouldn't that elicit a non-professional response? Aren't some people really not putting in their best effort to understand your child and his autism spectrum disorder? Does this mean you have to compromise every single time and never dig in your heels?

The answers are: Yes, no, yes, and certainly not.

There are times when the school system is so diametrically opposed to what you know to be right for your child's education that you must snort fire, spit nails, scream, kick (not other people), shout and otherwise make a spectacle of yourself. However, all other avenues should be exhausted before you make an emotional, immovable stand from which you will not be shaken.

"What you want is to be the parent they really don't want to deal with," one New Jersey mom told me. "If you go in with an attitude that you're not going to take anything from them, you'll see how far you can go."

The problem with a statement like that is that you don't want school personnel cringing when they hear your name; your phone call will be returned last, and the atmosphere before a meeting even begins will be one of contention and competition. What you really want is for the whole team, of which you are a part, to be working for the better education of your child, and sometimes that means being the parent they don't want to get mad.

How do you go about doing that? First of all, you have to spend time being the reasonable parent, the one who never comes in with Guns A' Blazing. My wife and I call ourselves the "good bagel parents" because we used to bring snacks to the IEP meetings we attended, until the school started putting out bagels and coffee for us.

Try to be the "good bagel parents" (or whatever kind of treat you prefer) for a while, especially when you're beginning the relationship with the school. Listen to everything that's said, never react emotionally or negatively, and while you don't have to agree with everything that's said, try not to be combative. Agree to think over any issues on which there's a disagreement. Don't sign an IEP you find inadequate or harmful, but keep offering your own versions in a calm, compromising way and see how that goes. Be personable with the school personnel. Talk to them about themselves, their background, anything that might help you understand their point of view better.

Make a sincere effort to keep everything, at worst, civil. Save your bullets for when you really need them.

When you've earned a reputation as the calm, reasonable "good bagel parent," don't start looking for an opportunity to let loose your frustration (if you have any). Continue to look for the best solution to each problem that everyone on the team can agree to implement.

But when the moment comes that an issue is not, in your opinion, negotiable, when your child's education or well-being is clearly on the line and you need to be the best advocate you can, that's the time to go in with Guns A' Blazing.

Because you will have spent so much time being a good team member, the other members (teachers, principal, etc.) will come to see you as an ally. So if the time comes that you have to be less conciliatory, the change in your demeanor will be much more effective.

Consider this: If two people at your place of business come to you with a problem, which would you consider more credible, the one who is constantly complaining about every detail of every transaction you make, or that one who is always easy to get along with, but now seems to be extremely upset about this one important issue? Which one would you help quicker? Which one would you work harder to please?

See my point?

There are times when it's important, even necessary, to express your displeasure with the solution (or lack thereof) to a problem offered by the school district. If there is no question that your child will not do well under the present circumstances, and that your solution is the only conceivable way to solve the problem, you have to become stubborn. You have to stop bringing the good bagels.

A word of warning, however: Sometimes pent-up emotion gets the better even of parents who have been calm and reasonable for months, or years. In fact, the amount of time that some parents feel they've been holding back is sometimes reflected in the vehemence with which they let go once they have a serious grievance.

One mother from New Jersey told me that her son had been so convinced his behavior was "bad" that "if someone raised their voice a little bit, he would jump into my lap and say, 'I'm sorry.'" These were parents who had been sure to "write thank-you notes when (the school district) did good things. We make sure the (school) board was cc'ed on those, because (the Child Study Team members) were really trying."

When the district dug in its heels and refused to budge on a diagnosis, however, she discovered that things weren't what she thought. "If there's one little problem you think you have, it's probably much larger than you think," she says now. "Now, the relationship is strained. This is their program, and they're not going to bend unless you hire an attorney. We complained, and went to court, and people were let go. They weren't following the IEP."

All that came about because the parents, who had been working well with the Child Study Team, showed their teeth when the issue was pressed and they felt it was important enough. The consequences were unusual, but their son is now in the proper environment in school, and doing well, working up to grade level.

Another New Jerseyan says her son was not doing well in a self-contained class, so she requested he be put into a mainstream class. "They said, 'we don't want (her son) to look different,'" she recalls. "I'm going along with this because I can be reasonable. He was getting along all right academically, but not with other kids."

Eventually, she appealed to her son's case manager, who was the school's social worker. "Between fourth and fifth grade, she figured him out," the mom recalls. "We started out as adversaries, but we ended up helping each other."

In this case, the parent and a member of the Child Study Team worked together to bring the problem to light. The mother's original attempt at dealing with the situation without becoming angry was unsuccessful, and becoming more vocal helped forge a bond with someone who had been working in another direction.

Even when you decide – and it must be a decision, not a reaction – to have your Guns A' Blazing, it's important to do so the right way. Whenever possible, keep it in writing. Avoid phone calls when the situation is serious, because there is no inherent proof that the conversation took place as either party will remember it. In writing, there is no such concern.

Also, keep it professional. Personal attacks, no matter what the circumstances are, will hurt your case. They'll also make it much more difficult to continue working with the people in your child's school who are, after all, the ones who see her on a regular basis.

Last, keep it an isolated incident. You can't make a habit of going ballistic; it will wear out its welcome very quickly, and stop being effective. You'll become the Parent Who Screamed Wolf. In order for such a tactic to work in any kind of negotiation, it has to be something that distinguishes itself because it's unusual.

Every parent of a child with special needs, such as those with disorders on the autism spectrum, reaches a point of frustration with schools on occasion. No one understands our children as well as we do, and we are given the added responsibility of understanding the disorder, something that not many teachers and school administrators can do as fully. It's easy to become frustrated and, in some cases, angry. But when we act on that emotion, we have to do so in a controlled, planned, calculated manner, in order to use it to our best advantage.

There's nothing wrong with going into a meeting with (proverbial) Guns A' Blazing, if that's something you've decided is necessary, and something you've planned ahead of time. If you're doing it as a reaction, as a response to something that struck an emotional chord with you, you will not be helping your child; you'll just be trying to make yourself feel better.

It's better to go to a gym and hit a punching bag for a while, if all you want to do is feel better. If you want to help your child get the best possible education, plan your outbursts, use them when you have to, and the rest of the time, keep those weapons in your holster.

It's not always easy to do, but it's the best possible strategy.

Chapter Twenty

TRANSITIONAL PRIMARY — A CASE STUDY FROM A VERY CLOSE VANTAGE POINT

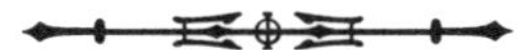

When our son was 4 years old, and we did not yet have a name for the differences we noticed in his behavior, he was enrolled in what was then called a "Pre-K Handicapped" program for children not yet in school, but whose entry into kindergarten appeared to be in jeopardy because of some disability. Josh did not yet have a diagnosis, other than that of a general "auditory processing" problem that wasn't really specified. It was roughly the third diagnosis we had been given at that point.

In the pre-Asperger days, the Pre-K program seemed to be the best option for a child who was having great difficulty relating to his peers, who tended to act out in the most socially unacceptable way he could find (Josh was a biter) and who really didn't seem to care much whether there were other children around or not. So he was enrolled. About four weeks went by with little word from the teacher or the school, both of whom were new to the program.

At the end of a month, we did receive a call from the school, the gist of which went something like this: "We don't see any problem with this child; please take him home."

Well, all parents want to hear that their child has no problems, so we were thrilled, took our son home and prepared for his entrance into kindergarten, only a few months away.

It was something of a surprise, therefore, when, about two weeks into Josh's kindergarten year, my wife was approached by his teacher when she was dropping him off one morning.

"There's a problem with your son," she said.

My wife was taken aback, since we'd been told by the school system less than six months earlier that there was no problem, and that our son would do very well in kindergarten. An academic problem? she asked.

"No. A behavior problem. He's not ready for school; you should probably wait a year before you try again."

This was a serious shock to our family. With a toddler of less than 2 years at home, we had been looking forward to the day we wouldn't have to pay for two children in day care. Worse, Josh had been desperate to go to school (a condition that alas, did not last, as is the case with most students as they get older), and would see any disruption of that routine as a punishment, a sign that he had done something wrong.

With the utmost respect, we had our first encounter with our district's school system. We told them that, since they had been the ones to tell us that kindergarten wouldn't be a problem for our son, we thought it would be their responsibility to make the situation work. We explained his state of mind, and suggested that sending Josh home from school would do more damage than it would do good.

To our great surprise, the school system – represented in this case by the teacher, the principal, the speech and language specialist and the social worker – agreed with our assessment. Josh stayed in kindergarten through the year, in the same class. And the teacher who had initially told us he wasn't ready for school became his greatest advocate, and our hero. When the class had a "graduation" ceremony from kindergarten, Josh gave her a huge hug, and the teacher almost broke down in tears; they were the best of friends by then.

The kindergarten year was not easy, however. Josh didn't like the feel of the wool rug on which the children sat for stories and other activities, and stood up or fidgeted during those times until he was allowed to sit elsewhere. He could rarely sit still anywhere in the room, was doing a lot of stimming, and seemed to have attention difficulties until asked about the lesson, when he would recite virtually verbatim what had been told to him. Finally, he didn't make much eye contact.

During that time, he was being evaluated by the Child Study Team, which included the school psychologist as well as the above-mentioned personnel. But no one had a definitive diagnosis for him until the Newgrange School of Hamilton, New Jersey (less than an hour from our home), held a seminar featuring members of the Yale Child Study program on a strange-sounding condition called Asperger Syndrome (AS).

My wife attended the all-day session, and by the time it broke for lunch, she had concluded that our son did indeed have Asperger's. To some degree, he exhibited virtually every behavior described at the seminar, and the description being given, as well as the videos of people with Asperger, matched him very closely. My wife got up from her seat at the lunch break and headed for the exit at the back of the room.

There stood our school psychologist, the speech specialist and the special education teacher. They stopped her as she left, and the conversation boiled down to an approximate, "aha!"

The diagnosis was confirmed very soon afterwards by a pediatric neurologist. Our son, then 5 years old, had Asperger Syndrome.

That didn't much change the rest of the kindergarten year. Josh had become ingrained enough in the daily routine that he could manage not to disrupt the class, and sometimes even participated in the lesson. He talked to the teacher, and sometimes to the other children in the class.

Near the end of the term, we were contacted about something that would become an annual ritual, our first IEP meeting. It was at that meeting that the idea of a transitional primary class was first broached.

As I've mentioned earlier, I was not immediately open to the prospect of our son putting off first grade for a year. Academically, he did not need any extra time; his work was very good, and he was learning all the basics children in kindergarten are expected to know. No one disputed that, but I felt that most of the children in the transitional primary class the following year would be there for academic help, while Josh needed social skills training. I had decided the school should provide that training, but the suggestion that an extra school year, between kindergarten and first grade, would provide that kind of help seemed excessive. Wouldn't he be falling a year behind the one or two friends he had managed to make in kindergarten? Wasn't that more damaging to his social skills and his self-esteem than what he might gain?

It was a critical point, as it was our first encounter with the school system at a moment when they were suggesting something we hadn't anticipated or requested. It sounded very much like the school was trying to get our son out of the way, out of the mainstream; excluded. We had heard the horror stories from other parents in the area, and were immediately wary.

But the arguments the teachers and specialists made were sensible ones: Josh's AS meant his emotional maturity was a little behind his chronological age, and the extra year would make great strides in bringing him even with the other children. And it would give the transitional primary teacher, who had a background in special education and a knowledge of what Asperger Syndrome was (something that was hard to come by in 1996), time to help him with social skills specifically, while getting him ready for the more structured environment that first grade would provide.

It took some time for us (okay, me) to come around, but we agreed to place Josh in Transitional Primary, and as I've said elsewhere in this book, it was probably the best decision we've made on his education to date.

The teacher, Lisa Bielen (now Lisa Capron), was perfect for the task – patient, young and enthusiastic – and Josh loved her. More important, she "got" Josh, understood his great strengths and areas of weakness, and knew how to build in him the skills he'd need to make it through a day with desks, sitting still, listening to a teacher talk, and dealing with other children. She helped him gain self-esteem by the bucketful, and prepared him for what was to come.

Time was the next most helpful factor. Given a year to develop his skills and a little maturity, Josh was better able to learn and play with other children when he had completed the transitional primary year. There were still problems with his social skills (some of which remain to this day, in a diluted and more mature form), but not nearly as many as there would have been if he'd immediately gone to first grade the year after kindergarten.

Also, because he was now a year older than most of his classmates, he was not as easy a target for bullies. Josh was bigger at 7 that he was at 6, and while he still took a good deal of teasing for his stimming and other "weird" quirks in the schoolyard, he was able to deal with the situation better than if he hadn't had the year to mature.

There were still problems in first grade, even with the extra year of school before it. Transitional Primary isn't a cure-all for autism spectrum disorders; it's simply one tool used to help our children cope with what's coming. Yes, there were still incidents of inappropriate behavior, especially in response to teasing, that continued for some time. At the end of second grade, Josh was given a full-time one-on-one aide, and he continues with her into his sophomore year of high school.

Transitional Primary did not make the Asperger Syndrome go away, and it never will. But it did provide help, and it was an experience that I believe has benefited my son in every grade since. It's not a solution, and it's not even a useful tool for every child on the spectrum, but in his case, that year made a large difference.

It also proved that a parent's initial reaction to a school system's suggestion need not be a contrary one, and that the first emotional response we have to anything related to our children's education need not be the impulse we always act upon. Sometimes, that first gut reaction is exactly right, and we should stick to our guns (pardon the expression) and refuse to be moved, but only when we've had the time to consider the situation, the reasons being given for the suggestion, and the impact it will have on our children, and not our own egos. We have to forget our own egos when we are acting as parents of children with autism spectrum disorders; they're irrelevant.

Even now, some 10 years removed from the class itself, Josh gets a particularly wistful look on his face when he's reminded of the transitional primary year. He met one of his closest friends in that class, and they remain friendly to this day, playing video games and clowning around in voices deeper than those of their fathers. And he enjoyed the time with a teacher who, in a class of smaller size, with a less jam-packed curriculum, managed to find more time for him than almost anyone else he has encountered in the school system.

It was a good year. Sometimes, I think it was his best year. I wish there had been another between middle school and high school; it would have made that transition a good deal easier.

Chapter Twenty-One

A DAILY VISIT TO THE NURSE

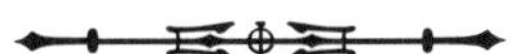

Not a terribly large number of years ago, Josh's pediatrician suggested that we try changing his medication. My son has been taking Ritalin since he was 6, and is still on a very low dosage. It helps him focus at school, and avoid frustration escalating into incidents that nobody finds pleasant.

Every day, Josh takes a 15 mg dose of Ritalin before leaving for school, then goes to the school nurse around the time he has lunch (usually at noon) each school day for another 10 mg. He's been doing this since he was in first grade.

The doctor's suggestion for a change in medication was a simple one: The new drug, Concerta, would be a longer-lasting medication that did the same job as the Ritalin, but would not require the dose at noon. So Josh could skip the trip to the nurse every day and, in theory, the teasing that went with such trips.

However, when we suggested the new pill to our son, he was confused as to why he would need it. We told him that he wouldn't need the Ritalin any more, that he could take one pill before he left for school, and that would be all for the day.

His eyes became wide and, I believe, a little damp. "But what about the trip to the nurse?" he asked. We told him that would no longer be necessary.

Josh absolutely refused. Medication is one thing, but eliminating the walk to the nurse's office every day was out of the question.

You can't ever tell with a child on the autism spectrum. When we asked, Josh explained that he liked the break in the middle of the day, he liked talking to the nurse, he didn't mind having to leave the lunchroom early, and the other kids never teased him about having to take medication in the middle of the school day. He explained it all in a tone that indicated we must be a little dizzy, even suggesting that he give up what he saw as a highlight in the school day.

Medication is a very personal issue with people on the autism spectrum. My wife and I have heard (quite vocally) from people who believe we are needlessly drugging our son, and others who believe he should be taking more medication. They seem to feel that discussing this subject with us, since we've been quite vocal about Josh's Asperger Syndrome, is perfectly acceptable and polite behavior. Frankly, I find it a little off-putting, but no two people react in exactly the same manner to anything, so I guess my response might not be anticipated.

My philosophy about Josh's medication has always been that it is a personal thing for him, and as his parents, we could make that determination when he was 6. Those who feel that any medication for autism is inappropriate should not medicate their children. Those who feel, as we do, that we've seen no negative side effects and that there is a benefit, should make the choice to do so. This book – and this chapter – are not about whether or not you should choose to give your child medication; that's your choice.

But for those of us who have decided that some medicine can help, the issue affects most aspects of our children's lives. We give Josh some "vacations" for his meds, when he's not in school or at camp and we have no plans that he might find stressful, because when he's relaxing, there's little need for it. When he's at school, however, it is important. Whenever he's forgotten to take his medication, or we've accidentally run out for a day, his aide immediately notices the change in his demeanor, and the added difficulty he feels getting through the school day.

At school, medication becomes a more public thing. Just because my son hasn't run into teasing because of his daily trip to the nurse doesn't mean others are exempt. One Oregon mother told me her son had tried Ritalin when younger, but found that the questions and the attention, which made him feel "different" than everyone else, overshadowed the benefit from the drug. Consequently, she and her husband decided to forego the medication, and her son was happier and more relaxed at school. There were still incidents and some difficulty with attention in class, but it was a question of degree, and the stress of the teasing had been worse than the lack of medication. That was their choice, and it worked out for their child.

Some school systems are not as helpful as others with medication. Legally, no school is allowed to deny a child the medication prescribed by a doctor and allowed by a parent or guardian, but some are more resistant than others, make the trip to the nurse more difficult than it should be (by trying to manipulate the time to accommodate the school schedule), or question – without denying the right – whether the medication is really necessary. One parent was told that the school would administer the medication as directed, but that the parent should "think about what you're doing to your child."

There's little a school system can do to stop you from giving your child medication, even if that takes place on school grounds. It's a little puzzling to even consider why schools would want to deter such a thing, as the aim of medication for children on the spectrum is either to ensure the child's health or to help the child get through a school day without incident. But some districts do seem to feel that it's an intrusion on the routine, an added burden for the school nurse, and a distraction to other children.

Again, I can't report any difficulties with my local school system on this topic, but a number of parents told me that the public schools their children attend have been less than cooperative about medication. More disturbing were the reports from parents that private schools – including one that caters to children with special needs! – were even more resistant to the idea of a child taking medicine for attention deficit disorder or related symptoms at school.

"They told me, 'it's our job to keep the children's attention,'" one mother from the Midwest said about the private school she interviewed as a possible placement for her child. "They said, 'we don't need the medication here.' I immediately crossed that school off my list."

There are rules that need to be obeyed with any medication, and with Ritalin, which is a controlled substance in most states, there are additional rules. My son may not medicate himself at school, despite his ability to do so quite effectively and responsibly at home. If the nurse runs out of pills, she may not simply call me and ask for more – they must be brought to school in the original pharmacy-issued bottle, or she isn't able to accept them. If Josh forgets to bring the bottle on the day it's required, I have to bring it to the school before he can return to class. It's a good thing I work at home, and am available most days, because his memory isn't always the best.

I appreciate the rules, and I don't fault the school for having to follow them. Again, part of keeping the blazing guns in my holster is understanding the school's point of view. They are not allowed, by law, to administer a controlled substance like Ritalin without following the state's guidelines for that substance. Josh understands it, and so do his parents. We follow the rules, and try to make the procedure as easy for the school nurse as it can be.

Through the years, Josh has known a different school nurse at three separate schools, and in some cases, more than one at each school (there is turnover in staff at any workplace). He is very personable when he decides to be, and the nurses have been his strongest advocates in the school, invariably, because they thoroughly enjoy seeing him and talking with him every day. He's never been a problem, never refused to take his medication, and often has new jokes to pass along whenever he stops by the nurse's office. Josh, without prompting, is learning to go in with no Guns A' Blazing, and that helps smooth the process.

Besides, as I noted above, he loves the break. When he was younger, he and Mrs. Gregus would go to the nurse's office together, but these days, Josh usually goes there on his own, and he appreciates the time alone. It doesn't hurt that the trip gets him out of the cafeteria, one of the most stressful places – loud noises, lots of people – in the school for my son.

There is no wiggle room on medication in schools. If you and your doctor decide that your child needs the meds, the school must allow for their administration. It's a no-compromise situation, and if the school flat-out refuses, you have no choice but to insist, and if necessary, to take legal action.

I've never heard of a school system refusing to give a child prescribed medication. They might not be thrilled about it, and in some cases try to dissuade parents, but even the most extreme cases never refuse to give a child medicine. For one thing, it's against the law.

The decision on medication is one of the most personal you will make for your child, and in some cases, with your child. Schools are not permitted to discuss your child's medication with anyone else unless they have your written permission. You can keep all word of any medicine your child receives private. However, the other children in the school will know that your child is going to the nurse for something every day, and there will be little question about what the reason is. Yes, there can be teasing, but with proper preparation, including a possible presentation as described in a previous chapter, the other students should understand. Not everyone will be kind, and there's nothing you can do about that, unfortunately.

The best thing to do is review your reasons for giving the medicine. If you believe you were right to do so, you have nothing to apologize for. If other students tease yours about having to take medication for an autism-related disorder, keep in mind that the medication is itself a tool to help your child deal with some of the stress – including teasing – that goes along with a normal school day for our children.

Nothing's easy for our children, and by extension, for us. The decision about and administration of medication is no exception. But with enough preparation and enough information, it doesn't have to be an unpleasant experience for your child.

Ask my son. He's already looking forward to his next visit to the nurse.

Chapter Twenty-Two

THE WORST TIMES OF THE DAY

For most children, school is a grind of lectures, class work and regimented routine, relieved only by the welcome change of pace that comes during recess (for younger students) and lunch (for everyone). During these times of the day, the structure is lifted, the children can socialize and play, and what seems like a boring, tedious, stressful day suddenly becomes an enjoyable respite that never seems to last long enough.

This is not true for our children.

For children with autism spectrum disorders, recess and lunch are usually the worst times of the day, fraught with stress, danger and uncertainty. For our routine-loving structure junkies, the prospect of spending time when there are few, if any, rules, when other kids will be loud and boisterous and may expect some social rituals that are hard to understand is positively frightening.

It's not easy to explain to parents whose children are neurotypical, and it's sometimes just as hard to make school systems understand, but our children would be much, much happier if recess and lunch were more like the rest of the day: in a quiet classroom, with strictly enforced rules and careful supervision from teachers who allow little, if any, talking among the students.

The horror stories that many parents tell involve times of the day when the children are relatively unsupervised and given more freedom to relax and "just be kids." The problem is that our children don't always know how to do that.

Quite often, a one-on-one aide for a child on the spectrum is most needed during the times when no academic work is being done. That's not always easy for a school district to understand, and it can lead to some disagreements and misunderstandings at IEP meetings and during the school year.

For teachers and those who don't "get" what spectrum disorders are like, the idea that a child needs more supervision and assistance during the "down" times in a school day is an indication that the child has "behavior issues," and not that he might simply be having trouble understanding what is expected of him during these times.

Anxiety isn't always visible is children with spectrum disorders. And even when it is, the heightened sense of unease usually looks more like anger or rudeness. So when children with spectrum disorders are presented with a situation that causes them to feel stress, they are not immediately perceived that way by people – including teachers – who are not familiar with autism and related disorders. This is especially true when the situation in question is not one that a neurotypical person would characterize as stressful.

I know of one boy, about 8, who had devised a ritual for himself that took the stress out of recess at his school. The problem was that, as with most children with spectrum disorders, his ritual chiefly involved the boy getting himself into a position where he would be assured of being left alone – atop a tire pile that served as playground equipment for his school.

That would have been a perfectly fine solution (albeit one that didn't advance the child's social skills in any way), if he hadn't chosen a spot that other children might occasionally like to visit. When that happened, the boy became very agitated, and occasionally hit or kicked children who tried to encroach upon what he saw as his territory.

The teachers assigned to that recess period were stumped for a solution to this problem, as banning the boy from his one spot would only escalate his sense of anxiety and probably cause more and more serious, incidents with other children. Eventually, it was decided, that for that particular recess period, every day, it would be made known that only this boy could play on this one particular pile of tires. The other children complied with the rule almost perfectly.

But the boy's father, who hadn't been notified about the new rule, but knew of the problems during recess, objected when he was told about the revised policy. His son shouldn't be rewarded for behaving inappropriately, he felt, and a general announcement to the class that the boy should be treated differently than everyone else wasn't going to help him learn social skills, and would make him seem more alien and scary to the other third graders. The father requested that the new policy be rescinded, that his son be told in no uncertain terms that he couldn't expect one section of the playground to be reserved for him, and that he would have to find another way to survive recess.

The school, in particular one teacher who did not have the boy in her class, resisted the suggestion. The boy with the spectrum disorder was not misbehaving any more, and the other children were content to leave him alone. As far as she was concerned, peace had been restored to the playground for the 30 minutes of recess the children had each day, so there was no reason to mess with success. But the boy's father was insistent: This policy, while it treated the symptom, in his eyes aided the disorder. His son would now believe that inappropriate behavior would help him get what he wanted and, worse, would be encouraged not to seek out other children to play with, but to become more withdrawn and not progress socially. The father believed that in this case, "tough love" was more appropriate than acquiescence. So he went into a meeting with Guns A' Blazing.

With two teachers who were assigned to the recess period and the principal, the father explained his disagreement with the solution the school had reached for his son's problem. The teachers explained that it was now much easier for them to maintain some order during recess, that the policy seemed to be working, and that everyone – especially his son – seemed content.

"In fact, they told me that I was the only one who wasn't getting with the program," the father told me. "I think they were starting to understand where (my son's) behavior had come from."

It never got to the point that the father had to threaten court action or hire an advocate, but the meetings did get to be contentious, he says. Eventually, more than a month after the teachers had started the "reserved" policy, the father's point of view prevailed, and the boy was told that he couldn't expect "his" tire pile to be exclusively his any more.

But the teachers made the father tell the boy himself. They backed up the information when the boy asked, but they wouldn't initiate the conversation.

"I don't think they ever really understood what I was getting at," the father says now. "I think I got my way the same way (my son) got his way – by not allowing them to say no."

It's not difficult to understand a school's desire for order on the playground, but it is a problem when order becomes more important than the needs of any one child in the class. In this case, the school addressed the issue by sidestepping it, giving the child an accommodation that hadn't been requested and shouldn't have been offered, in order to maintain some kind of calm during a recess period. The teacher's point of view – that the boy wouldn't be helped by being disciplined for something that was relieving his stress – was laudable, but the proposed solution was not a good one. It would only have encouraged the boy to hold out for an accommodation every time he didn't like the way something at school was organized and, eventually, that would have led to much larger problems.

The lunchroom, where many of us spent some rough times in school (particularly as we got a little older and cliques started), is even more difficult for children with spectrum disorders. In many cases, they have sensory issues that most neurotypical children do not have: Smells are more intense; the sight of people eating is disturbing for many children on the spectrum, and that's just the beginning.

Noise is almost always an issue. Crowds (except in the smallest schools) can be disturbing. There isn't much that lunchtime has to recommend itself for a child with a spectrum disorder, and that often includes the food itself.

Many of our children have food-related issues. My son is still considered a "picky" eater, although he has progressed considerably since he was younger. Others are much more rigid in their food choices, and often will not eat anything that is served in a school cafeteria. Worse, they often won't eat anything that can be realistically imported from home, and therefore refuse to eat lunch in school at all.

Some parents have asked for accommodations to allow their children to eat lunch at home, but that's not logistically possible for parents who work outside the home, or for those who live too far from the school to make it back and forth in the allotted time.

In some cases, parents have asked for – and gotten – permission for their children to eat lunch outside the main cafeteria, which makes the noise, the crowds and the olfactory issues less difficult. But some parents don't want their children, autism or not, to be excluded from the group during this extremely social time, and even when they do, exclusion from the lunchroom does not address the issue of a portable, palatable lunch.

With children on the spectrum, particularly those on the more high-functioning end, preparation is everything. If the child can be adequately prepared for what lunch will be like in a school – for example, if a child who will attend the school beginning the next term can be brought in for a visit ahead of time to see the situation, much progress can be made toward helping ease the anxiety. But the loud room, crowds and other distractions could just as easily heighten the child's worries, making the visit ahead of time an experience that will build anxiety for the entire summer until school begins again.

There's no one simple solution to the problem, as there is no one way to deal with all children on any issue. You know your child's culinary choices best. With a good deal of talk ahead of time, you and your child might be able to find an acceptable lunch, either bought at school or brought from home. Be warned, though, that one menu item might be all the child will be willing to eat for years on end. It took quite some time before my son would expand his horizons beyond one acceptable lunch.

If you feel a removal from the lunchroom is the best way to keep your child calm, perhaps you should request an alternate location – a classroom, the nurse's office or another room – where your child can have lunch. It won't improve his social skills, but sometimes a parent of a child on the spectrum has to choose which battle to fight while putting off the rest for a while.

All of this should be discussed with your child ahead of time whenever possible, and then broached with teachers and school personnel. There's no sense in fighting tooth and nail over something with the school, receiving it, and then discover that your child refuses to comply with the accommodation you've requested. Over the years, I've anticipated my son's reaction to something and been surprised – sometimes pleasantly – by his real response too many times to think I hold all the answers before the questions are asked.

Lunch and recess are the worst times of the day. But keep this in mind – in his freshman year of high school, my son had assembled a group of friends (a small one, I'll grant you) and they ate lunch at the same table every day. He would often come home and tell me about the conversations. Josh really seemed to enjoy that time.

Go figure.

Chapter Twenty-Three

IRRETRIEVABLE LOSS

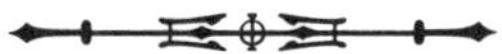

For six summers, my son attended a day camp about 45 minutes from our home called Harbor Haven, a place specifically designed for children with some social and neurological disorders, particularly Asperger Syndrome and attention deficit hyperactivity disorder. This happened after Josh was asked to leave a day camp for neurotypical children because the staff felt they "couldn't handle" him.

We were very pleased with the staff at Harbor Haven, and believe the care and attention he received there helped Josh in his social skills development. He made some good friends at the camp, and an academic component it offered, coupled with some social skills training, occupational therapy and other services, made it easier for Josh to transition from grade to grade as he went through school.

Because Harbor Haven insists on hiring counselors and staff who are well trained in the educational and neurological conditions with which they will be dealing, and because of geographical and other concerns, tuition at the camp is high. There were summers when it was difficult for us to pay the bill, but it was always paid. We felt that because of the type of training being given to Josh at the camp, and because of the construction of his IEP, we might expect to ask the school district for some assistance in sending him there.

My wife and I were not trying to "milk" the school system, to get them to pay for something that was not within their area of concern. Joshua always had a difficult time transitioning to a new year of school; his grades were always lowest in the first marking period, and most of his "meltdowns" or incidents that caused him trouble occurred during the first month or two of the school year. After he began attending Harbor Haven, and his social skills training and other services were reinforced during the summer, he found it less difficult to begin a new school year, and although fall was still his least successful semester, there was definitely improvement in his grades and behavior.

So we felt that, given Josh's change in performance as a result of attending the camp, and because he clearly needed help during the summer to maintain his academic and social development, our local school system might see the benefit of the camp and help with a specific percentage of the tuition that was devoted to the therapies and training (we did not expect the school system to pay for swim lessons or softball games).

The school system, for the first time since we had started dealing with them, said "no."

Summer, like recess and lunch, is an unstructured time. It's the time of year when children are supposed to be able to relax, to "just be kids," and to play and enjoy the outdoors. For many of our children, for whom a lack of structure is a terrifying concept, summer is a 10-week recess period, and that's decidedly not a good thing for them.

For many children with autism spectrum disorders, summer is a time when they have to learn new names, play games in which they hold no interest, learn new routines that don't match the old ones, participate in activities they might find frightening or uninteresting, and lose the momentum they had established during 10 long months in school.

It is not unusual for children with spectrum disorders to experience difficulties during the summer that carry over into the following school year. The lack of continuity in routine can cause what school officials call an "irretrievable loss," an academic erosion that occurs when the child doesn't "flex his muscles" in that area for an extended period of time, like during a long school vacation or summer break. Grades suffer, problem behavior often follows, and the child has to re-learn many concepts, both course-related and otherwise, that she had already mastered at the end of the previous school year.

The solution to such a problem is the Extended School Year (ESY), which most children would consider a punishment but children with spectrum disorders quite often think is a reward. ESY, connected either to the child's school or in a separate facility, extends the school year through the summer. It doesn't necessarily continue every part of a typical school day, but the program usually strives to refresh the child's memory of the academic subjects she takes during the year, and also the routine of a school day, as well as the social aspects that often cause serious difficulty for our children.

Sometimes, ESY can be a godsend; other times, the program offered by the local district is not geared toward autism spectrum disorders, and therefore may end up doing more harm than good.

In our case, in declining to pay for the parts of the Harbor Haven day that pertained to social skills or academic training, or to occupational or other therapies, the school district offered a program that was an academic program provided mostly for children who had been having trouble with their academics (Josh had not). We felt the program was inappropriate for our son.

It was, I reiterate, the first time we had come into serious disagreement with the local school system, which had been extremely helpful and cooperative until that point. And I understood the point they were trying to make: The law states that a program needs to be in place that is adequate to the student's needs, not one that is the best and most complete therapy indicated for the student. Once again, it was the distinction between what gives the child the chance to have the same education as neurotypical children and what gives him an unusual advantage.

We came down on the side of equality, and the school saw it as an extraordinary accommodation.

We pulled those long-forgotten pistols out of the closet and reholstered them, and went to many a meeting. I remember arguing that the school was waiting for Josh to fail before it would help him, and that I saw the camp as a way to prevent failure. Voices were raised, but not in anger, and no personal remarks were exchanged. There was no bad blood, but we were disappointed that the school wouldn't see our side of the issue, or at least, was not willing to acquiesce to it.

The disagreement ended up in a state mediation, a step we had never considered before, and have had no reason to consider since. The outcome seemed predetermined, the day was not pleasant, and we walked out with a decision from the mediator that was not the one we had hoped for.

Frankly, time had become an issue: It was spring, and Josh had to be enrolled in Harbor Haven before all the spaces were filled. We knew that other parents whose children were in the camp under similar circumstances had received financial aid from their school systems without the mediation, and we were disappointed.

The decision now was whether to continue with a due process hearing, which would take more time (and seemed to have just as predetermined an outcome), or moving on. We moved on. Josh attended camp for one more summer (his last there, because of age restrictions), and we found a way to pay his tuition again.

Extended School Year programs range widely from simple academic "reminders" that help students keep a grasp on the material they've learned throughout a school year, and those that consist of every possible tool, including ABA, occupational therapy, speech and language instruction, social skills training and any number of other services. Each district will have a separate program (and some have no program at all), and as we discovered, finding out about it in plenty of time is key.

At your child's IEP annual meeting, the issue of ESY is almost certain to be raised, if for no other reason than because many states require it. Even if you don't believe your child needs an extended program, at least investigate what is included in the local ESY plan. As your child grows, you might find it to be a useful tool.

If you feel that your child would benefit from ESY, begin discussing it as early as possible. Find out about the school district's program, and be ready with suggestions (not requirements) of what your child might require. If the program already includes provisions that you think will help your child, you're one step ahead of the game. If it doesn't, you have time to request them, or to find alternative – possibly out-of-district – programs that do.

Obviously, I can't guarantee that you'll find the perfect ESY program for your child, or that your child will benefit from any such plan. But planning ahead, having experts evaluate your child's strengths and weaknesses to your satisfaction, and determining what kind of extended program would be of the most help to your child can't hurt, and should be done within the school system.

"We had never even considered Extended School Year before the school brought it up at an IEP meeting, and I don't think they really thought it was a good idea," says one Nebraska mom. "I think they had to mention it, so they mentioned it. But our son (who has Asperger Syndrome) is so set on going to school every day that just being in the building during the summer was going to help him, and when we suggested it to the (special education teacher), I have to say, she immediately agreed it was a good idea. He's been in the program for two summers now, and he's never lost at sea when school starts again, like he used to be."

My own son's experience with ESY never gelled. Summer camp – even a special needs summer camp – isn't what the ESY laws have in mind, and what the local district was offering was not what Josh needed. But he comes through summer pretty well now as he's just about to turn 16, and hopefully from now on, he'll be able to avail himself of a completely different kind of "extended school year": A summer job.

Chapter Twenty-Four

TESTS, AND HOW TO PASS THEM

There is a fine distinction between learning the material being taught in school and being able to pass a test on the material being taught in school. Many children are perfectly capable of learning what is being taught, but have difficulty demonstrating that knowledge on paper, especially on a form created for a standardized test.

Welcome, once again, to the world of children with disorders on the autism spectrum.

Tests are a distinct difficulty for many children who have spectrum disorders for a number of reasons. The disruption of a school routine to take a test, for one, will put some of our children off their game to begin with. And some, like my son, are indifferent to their grades, so tests don't mean that much to them.

Other children with disorders on the spectrum have difficulty understanding the instructions, or lack the fine-motor skills necessary to blacken only one small spot on a standardized test with a No. 2 pencil.

Enter the IEP. Provisions can be written into a personalized education program that will level the playing field for children with spectrum disorders, and they should be discussed and customized to your child's needs at the annual IEP meeting, or at any time you or the school feels a revision to the existing document is necessary.

"My son couldn't possibly take tests – especially the statewide standardized tests – without his aide and without someone to make the marks on the paper in the right place," says one mother in Ohio. "They have to be carefully monitored so that it's clear they're making the marks where (my son) tells them to, and not helping him with the answers, but otherwise, his fine-motor skills just wouldn't allow him to get through the test in the time they give you."

Another common accommodation is to allow the child, if motor skills difficulties or other physical disabilities make writing difficult, more time than is typically allotted to take a test. In some cases, computer keyboards can be substituted for pencil and paper, particularly if there is a good deal of writing (an essay, for example) involved in the test.

The accommodations you feel are necessary to make test-taking possible for your child must be included in the IEP document before the testing is to take place. This year, since our son will be taking his PSATs in his sophomore year of high school, we were very careful to ask for accommodations on time and motor skills, even though we are relatively sure Josh won't need them. They are a safety net, available in case the experience turns out to be more than he can handle. If not, he is under no requirement to take extra time or type on a computer when the test requires written words.

As usual, our school system did not balk at the idea that Josh might require extra help; in fact, as I recall it, the subject of accommodations for standardized tests was broached by the school, not by us. We probably would have asked for the same supports, but we didn't need to ask, as they were being suggested on our son's behalf by a member of the Child Study Team.

Again, a number of private and public school systems will not be equally accommodating. In fact, the suggestion that a child needs extra help on tests of any kind can spark some serious arguments and cause many a gun to go a' blazing.

"We knew (our son) couldn't possibly manage to take the SATs without some kind of help," says one mother from New Hampshire. "The school thought we were trying to get 'an edge' on the test; they thought we were trying to make sure our son would do better than all the other kids in his class. What we were trying to do was to make sure he had a chance to do as well as he could, given how well he knew the things he was being tested on."

Several good arguments can be made on behalf of a child with an autism spectrum disorder and his need for some accommodations on tests, but in order to formulate the most effective defense, we must understand what the offense is going to be, and how it is motivated. Why would a school try to stop a child from doing as well as possible on a test?

Naturally, the school will not see things that way. Many parents who have requested IEP listings of extra help on tests say their districts chafe at the idea that a child is being given "an extra tool," that he will have "an unfair advantage," and that the school's responsibility is to every child "and not just your son (or daughter)."

It's necessary to keep an eye on your blood pressure when such statements are made, because reacting the way you want to will not help your child's case. We are not trying to "cheat the system" and give our children an unfair advantage. Our position should be that our children are currently at an unfair disadvantage if the rules are obeyed to the letter, and in order to give them a fighting chance to score as well as their natural abilitie sallow, they need a few accommodations that will make the test as hard for them as it is for other children and not harder.

This argument – that children with spectrum disorders will do too well on tests if they are given more time or other help – is usually proffered by teachers and others who don't truly understand the disorder (see Chapter Eighteen), and think we and our children are truly attempting to "scam" the educational system to achieve an unfair advantage. It's rarely helpful to try and convince people who are that closed-minded. Often the best tactic is to find someone else, preferably someone with more authority on the subject, to talk to.

Better, and better advised, is to appeal to what increasingly drives a school and its representatives: Better standardized test scores throughout the district mean better chances at state and federal funding, and increase the prestige of the school system as a whole.

This is why it always amazes me when school districts are eager to send children with autism spectrum disorders out of district because they think those children will hurt the district's overall rank. I know of at least one district that is willing to spend more than $30,000 a year to bus a child to a private school for students with special needs, based (according to one teacher) on the district's desire to keep test scores high rather than on the child's overall disability and his need for extra help.

Our children are not impaired academically; they are capable of just as much, if not more, than most neurotypical children. Studies suggest that children on the higher functioning end of the spectrum have, on average, higher IQ scores than the mean, and that would translate into higher scores on standardized tests and better overall rankings for school districts that include such children. If those districts allow for a few accommodations that may help children on the spectrum take tests more easily and unleash the knowledge they have accumulated in school and out.

People with a taste for kitschy nicknames sometimes refer to Asperger Syndrome as "The Little Professor Syndrome" because our children often latch onto one subject, learn everything there is to know about it, and then make a point of passing on that knowledge to anyone who will sit still long enough to listen. If that depth of accumulated facts can be allowed to run free on the pages of a standardized test, will the scores be higher or lower than we might expect?

So, appealing to the part of a school system that wants higher overall scores and, therefore, better ranks in the county, state, country or region is a strong tool to use in trying to get the accommodations your child might need written into an IEP. Let the teachers know that a laptop computer, rather than a clumsy hand, might help the school rise above a neighboring community in test scores, and watch that person's eyes light up. It's a base emotion to appeal to, but it can work.

Of course, you might not run into any opposition on the subject; many school districts are more than happy to help a child do better, and will suggest changes to the IEP that can do so. Also, we must make sure that we really aren't asking for an "edge," since the world of standardized testing, particularly at the high school level, has become incredibly competitive. It's tempting to ask for something you child might not need, but could use to increase his chances of getting good scores, but we have to resist that temptation. For one thing, such special help probably wouldn't do that much good anyway, and it will be questioned. Teachers and professionals who have tested your child will know if you're asking for an unreasonable accommodation. Most parents in our position don't do that, and for good reason.

Besides extra time and electronic keyboards, it is possible to request that your child be given tests in a separate room, if noise or crowding are especially distracting to her. You can also request that some parts of the test be taken orally, if your child has difficulty writing or filling in standardized test answers. These are completely legitimate accommodations that have been given to many children across the country (and around the world) who need help because of autism spectrum disorders and similar challenges.

Think about the ways your child's disorder manifests itself. What about particular quirks that might have an impact on the way he takes tests? What would make a difference in the test score? Those are the issues you need to address in the IEP.

An IEP is not a multiple-choice quiz. You don't have to choose from a list of standard accommodations and plug in the ones that fit. It's a chance to be creative. If your child has an issue that no child has voiced concerns about before, there's no reason not to address it, if it will make a serious difference in your child's success at school, particularly on tests.

As ever, the key is to have a smooth working relationship with the members of your school system's Child Study Team. If you've established yourself as reasonable and flexible, you should encounter fewer problems with testing than in other areas of IEP negotiation. Teachers, after all, do want their students to do well, and tests are the barometer we use to measure students' success.

There's no reason to be nervous about testing. After all, you've probably already taken your SATs. Keep working hard at helping your child with an autism spectrum disorder, and you'll pass any test you set up for yourself.

Chapter Twenty-Five

HOMEWORK

We decided to tell my son about his Asperger Syndrome when he was 8 years old. My wife and I believed that he was old enough to understand most of what it meant, and it would serve to explain why some of the other children in his class might be teasing him about behavior he saw as quite logical, or ignored completely.

I remember rehearsing ahead of time what I'd say to Josh, beginning with, "there's nothing wrong with you." I went on to tell him that he had something called Asperger Syndrome, and that while he wasn't in the least bit sick, it meant that his brain worked a little differently than most people's brains work. I told him that he would always have AS, but that he could be taught things in different ways that would help him understand what other people picked up naturally.

Josh took it all in, didn't seem upset, and finally went back to whatever it was he had been doing.

The next day, he came home with an unusually large pile of books under his arm. "Boy, I have a lot of homework today," he complained, then gave me a quizzical look. "How much of it do I have to do?"

That probably drew an equally quizzical look from me. "What do you mean, how much?" I asked. "You have to do all of it, just like always."

Now his face took on the appalled look of a person who has just been told that everybody gets ice cream but him. "But my brain works differently!" he shouted.

When people ask me to explain what children with Asperger Syndrome are like, I usually try to beg off, explaining that each child is different, that some are more affected than others, and various similar dodges. If they press on, I usually say that kids with AS are just like all other kids – only more.

That said, almost any child hates the idea of homework; it eats into their play time and continues the part of the day when they feel most put-upon. So if almost all children hate homework, it follows that children who have autism spectrum disorders hate it too – only more.

The most serious, unpleasant battles we ever had in my house were the ones revolving around Joshua's homework when he was in early grades of school – ironically, when the homework was simplest and could be done most quickly. Josh insisted on relaxing when he got home from what we were sure was a stressful day of trying to "fit in" with the neurotypical children. As the parent who mans the fort (that is, the house) for after-school activities, I relented, feeling that with a little battery recharging, he'd be able to attack the homework assignments with a clearer head and a more positive attitude.

I couldn't have been more wrong.

Breaking from the routine of the day, getting out of the school mindset, was the worst possible thing for Josh when he got home from school. Because he was able to do most of the homework relatively easily, he could have finished most days' homework in a very short time, often under 30 minutes, almost always in less than an hour. But since he was so adamant about needing time to play after school, my wife and I agreed that he do his homework after dinner.

It never went well. First, it was difficult to get Josh to even take out the worksheets and look at what had to be done. Then, he'd immediately conclude that the work was "too hard," that it would take "too long," and that (and all this is in the course of less than a minute) he "couldn't do it."

His bedtime was a lot earlier in those days, and he still needed to bathe and do a few things that made up his nighttime ritual. There was not enough time for a tantrum and homework, but that was very often what happened in our house. Josh had convinced himself that there was no point to trying, as he could not do the work assigned, concluding that the teacher would simply have to understand the next day that the assignment was an unreasonable one.

Screaming, crying and yelling ensued, and Josh behaved badly, too.

After a period that I'm sure wasn't as long as it seemed, my wife and I finally realized what we should have seen from the start: The delay between arriving home from school and doing the homework assignment was the problem. If Josh came home still in a "school" state of mind, and immediately got to work on what he had to do, he would have the rest of the day to do what he wanted. Maybe that would make a difference in his attitude.

The first hurdle was selling this plan to my son. I made a point of talking to him as soon as he arrived home from school one day. I explained why we thought this would work better, emphasizing that after he had done his homework, he wouldn't have to think about it for the rest of the day. Then I told him that the new plan wouldn't go into effect until the next day, to give him time to think about it.

"No," he said, "I think I'll try it now."

He did his homework right after school that day, and has been doing so since then. He's 16 years old now, so the tantrums are not the problem they used to be. Josh's anxiety level regarding homework is definitely lower than it was when he was younger. He's still not crazy about it, but he doesn't question when it needs to be done any more, and even if it takes longer than it used to, he keeps at it until it's done.

Projects and reading assignments are another story, but this is a book, not an encyclopedia.

One thing schools and teachers are adamant about is homework, and it's easy to understand why. I've taught classes myself, and I know that homework is probably the best way to see if a student is grasping the material as the course goes on, to identify problems, or students who might need extra help before the situation gets out of hand. So homework is not something that we as parents of children with spectrum disorders should be trying to eliminate.

On the other hand, our kids are not your standard-issue children, either, and they have special concerns when it comes to continuing the school day into the time spent at home.

Schools and parents don't often come into conflict over the concept of homework. But the amount of it, and the manner in which it is assigned and expected to be completed, can be the source of disagreement. While these issues rarely take on the scope of placement questions or diagnosis disagreements, they can have an effect on the child's school years.

For our son, as an example, long-term projects were always a problem. Josh treated them like he did his regular homework, and often tried to put off doing the work until the day before the project was due. I confess that sometimes I didn't pay enough attention to when assignments were due, having already graduated fourth grade myself. However, we were unable to convince our son that doing the work in increments was the way to tackle a project.

With help from his teachers and the Child Study Team, however, we worked out a solution. Part of Josh's IEP now reads that long-term projects should be assigned in increments, with specific due dates, so that Josh understands each piece of the assignment, and when he's expected to have it done. It's not a perfect system, but it resulted from cooperation between the parents (that's us) and the school system.

Other parents have not had it so easy. One mother from Massachusetts told me that her son's teacher couldn't understand why the boy wanted to type assignments on the home computer and print them out, even though she had seen that fine-motor skills deficiencies made his handwriting almost illegible. "She had seen his classwork," the parent marveled. "She knew how hard it was, and how long it took him, to write something in longhand. If it had been an assignment in handwriting, I could understand it, and he was getting (occupational therapy) for his motor skills, which she knew. But she kept complaining, saying she wasn't sure whether the work was (her son's) or whether someone at home was helping him."

Eventually, the principal interceded and took the side of the parents. As a result, the boy was allowed to submit assignments that had been printed on a home computer. Once again, the level of understanding among people who should have been trained in the areas of special education and inclusion (the teachers) worked against the boy with a spectrum disorder.

More often, disagreements come up about the amount of homework being assigned. Some parents believe children with spectrum disorders should not be required to do as much homework as their peers, particularly anything that requires a large amount of writing, while others, whose children are more high functioning and may be in the gifted category, feel their children are not being challenged enough, and in some cases, demand more homework.

If you are considering any of these options, the best thing to do first is to observe your child doing homework and see what happens when the homework is corrected and returned. If there is a noticeable pattern of difficulty for your child, or if certain types of items (arithmetic problems, creative writing assignments) aren't being done on a consistent basis, you might consider talking to your child, and then to his teacher.

But the way your child does homework is going to be much more grounded in your domain than the teacher's. For our son, the timetable was central: He had to do his work as soon as he got home, and not later. For other children, the area of difficulty may be in relation to blood sugar levels, which would mean a snack before homework, or relate to certain subjects, which might require help from one parent or another who might have more expertise (my wife is the math person, and I do English; we're both useless in science).

Homework is the area of the school day in which parents have the most control and the most influence. We need to see things that way in order to do the best job we can in making the experience workable for our children, spectrum disorder or not.

Keep this in mind: Your child is probably never going to like homework, no matter what. With that as a basis, you can handle whatever might come. It's a question of how much children don't like it, what will make them willing to do it (rewards, emphasis on report cards, blackmail) and taking the time – and this can be tough for parents – to help when the help is needed. I know that working at home makes me a little testy when I'm on a deadline and one of my children asks for homework help, but I have to remind myself that my first responsibility is to them. So I take a deep breath and lend a hand whenever I'm able.

After all, I'm just like any other father – only more.

Chapter Twenty-Six

HOW COME HE'S GETTING ALL THE ATTENTION?

A friend of mine teaches a class to nursing students at a local university. On occasion she has asked me to give a guest lecture on Asperger Syndrome and related disorders, particularly aimed at those of her students who plan to work as school nurses after graduation.

After one of the lectures recently, when I was taking questions, one of the students asked about my daughter, who is three years younger than her brother, and neurotypical. "Does she feel that she hasn't gotten the same amount of attention that your son does?" the student asked.

I answered that we have been very careful to make sure my daughter knows that we care as much about her as we do about Josh, and we have been diligent about attending every play, every graduation, every presentation she has been involved with. We pay attention to her interests and her personality, so I was sure she didn't feel deprived.

When I arrived home from the lecture that night, I told my daughter about the question and about the answer I'd given. She immediately gave me a look that indicated that my response might not have been correct. "You do feel we don't give you enough attention?" I asked, frankly a little amazed.

"I used to," she answered, "but mostly at school."

Why would she feel that way at school? "Well, Josh gets to go to OT, and he gets to go to speech therapy, and I have to go to math," she explained.

You can't please all of the people all of the time.

At some point, neurotypical siblings of children who have spectrum disorders, inevitably, feel that they are the forgotten children, the ones who don't get as much parental and school attention because, well, they don't seem to need it. Quite often that's not the truth, however. The neurotypical child does get just as much attention as his sibling with a spectrum disorder, but try to tell that to a younger or older sibling when he's feeling neglected.

In school, the problem is compounded. The neurotypical child might be teased for behavior her brother exhibited. She might be identified by teachers and administrators as "(the other child's) sister," rather than as an individual. She might even have to endure a move from one home to another because a different school district might be more accommodating to children with special needs, and have to sacrifice her friends and her home in the service of another child in the family.

"We had two years of hell," one Minnesota woman told me. "It was tearing our family up." Her children endured more than one move before she invoked the state's program that allows parents one choice of a school district. The change, despite uprooting the family, has proved beneficial. "I have two daughters and a son, and they are all wonderful with (her son on the spectrum)," she says.

Some siblings are not as forgiving. In some cases, they resent the intrusion on their lives, the added responsibility, the time taken away from their parents, that go along with having a sibling with a disorder on the autism spectrum. For younger children, especially, it's difficult to understand why a parent can't come to the dance recital or the ballgame because it's time for social skills group or occupational therapy. Similarly, when a child with a spectrum disorder must be home schooled, the siblings might not prefer to be taken out of the local system, or might wish to be, but parents can almost be assured that whichever decision they make will be seen as the wrong one.

Sibling rivalry is natural and, as with most other natural things, is amplified in a home with a spectrum disorder. From a child's point of view, it's easy to see how someone who is constantly getting away with infractions that would be considered unacceptable by a neurotypical child, someone who is always being driven to one appointment or another, someone whose tiniest step forward is hailed as momentous, might be a source of some resentment.

In my family, we have tried to treat our children equally, but that's never possible, even with two neurotypical children. Personalities require specific accommodations. When a spectrum disorder enters the mix, the accommodations become more frequent and more noticeable, and children, who are constantly searching for evidence that they are being slighted, become convinced that the scales are tipped in the wrong direction.

"(His older brother) really doesn't talk to (her son with autism) any more," says one Connecticut mother of teenagers. "He got it in his head at some point that (his brother) was getting better treatment, and that was it."

There's no simple solution to this problem, other than to try your best to show as much affection and attention to neurotypical siblings as to the child who has a spectrum disorder. Convincing all the children they are being treated equally is probably a waste of time, but through your actions, you can at least point to times spent with each one. Always be there for the important milestones, and if the neurotypical sibling is having difficulties at school or with something at home, lend as much support as you would to any of your children.

At school, the situation can become more complicated. Classmates may tease your child with the spectrum disorder, but that will filter down (or up, as the case may be) to your neurotypical children as well, and that's a very difficult position for a sibling to be thrust into. On the one hand, older siblings especially feel obligated to defend their brother or sister, but they may also be embarrassed by some of the behavior the child with the disorder exhibits, and that can be hard to defend.

Also, the teasing can go beyond comments about the child with a spectrum disorder to become more personal, tying your neurotypical child to the disorder, rather than the sibling. When a young child, especially, is forced to defend himself against comments that he is "different," that can be very stressful for everyone in the family.

Antagonism among the children can occur, as the neurotypical sibling believes she is being persecuted because of an "accidental" familial association. Add to that the possibility that the child has already felt neglected because of the extra attention the spectrum disorder demands, and you have a recipe for a very difficult family dynamic.

The first thing to do is to work through the school. Contact any teachers involved, and if they haven't already seen it, give them the Tips for Teaching document I included in Chapter Eighteen or something similar you have found that works. Explain the situation, and ask for some sensitivity. Most teachers will be happy to talk to the students involved, but that doesn't always make the difference.

In some cases, getting to know the parents of the children who are doing the teasing might help. As with any such situation, parents should know when their children are treating someone else badly, and in some cases, it's possible they'll be able to stop the behavior by talking to their children. But it's always potentially dangerous to bring authority figures – parents or teachers – into the situation with bullies, because they generally find a way to continue the bad behavior, but avoid getting caught, a skill a child with an autism spectrum disorder – due to inherent characteristics – rarely manages to develop.

The "dog-and-pony" show approach mentioned in Chapter Sixteen might be a valuable tool here. Children who understand spectrum disorders are more tolerant than those who are not informed. The presentation, whether by a parent, a teacher or an expert, should not be limited to the class that contains the child with the disorder. It should at the very least also include the classes of the child's siblings, and ideally, should be shown to everyone in school old enough to understand it.

"We showed it to everyone in the middle school," one Illinois parent says of a video that explains and illustrates Asperger Syndrome. "My daughter (with AS) benefited from it, but so did my son, who's two years older and doesn't have (a spectrum disorder). After that, his friends told him they understood what his sister was about."

Siblings in school often try as hard as they can not to notice each other, but children with spectrum disorders often don't pick up those social cues. They'll spot a brother or sister across a crowded hallway and call out, breaking one of the cardinal rules of pre-teen and teenager life: Don't draw attention to yourself.

While children with spectrum disorders can be taught not to yell across a hall to their siblings, they might not understand why they're being asked to do so, and can come to the conclusion that their siblings don't like them, or are ashamed of them. You can't force words into your children's mouths, but you can impress upon all your children the importance of understanding and fair treatment of others.

When the neurotypical siblings point out the "preferential" treatment being given their brother or sister, you might note that the child complaining can already interpret body language, tone of voice and make eye contact, that they can tell what someone means when he says he's "pulling your leg," and that they probably can hold a pencil properly after the age of 6. In short, there's no reason for them to feel sorry for their sibling on the spectrum, but there's no reason to feel inferior either.

The first time we took Josh to see the Harbor Haven Day Camp, where he would spend a number of summers with other children who had a neurological disorder that affected their behavior, we went as a family. We hadn't decided this would be the place for our son to relax during the summer, but we had a good idea that it would suit him.

And it did; there were baseball fields and a large swimming pool. We were pleased to hear that there would be social skills instruction and some academics, that disputes between campers were quickly resolved by a counselor who was trained in that area, and that if Josh needed occupational therapy or speech instruction during the summer, it was possible to find those things at the camp as well.

Our children saw mostly the swimming pool and the tennis courts. When we were preparing to drive home after the tour, Josh was his normal quiet self, preferring to keep his thoughts to himself, and probably concentrating on his GameBoy in the back seat of the car. My wife and I exchanged glances that indicated we were in agreement on the camp, and that we had reached a positive decision.

My daughter, all of 6 years old at the time, looked out the back window as we drove away, and in a clear, loud voice announced, "Daddy! I want to go to Asperger camp, too!"

Alas, she had to make do elsewhere. But she's gotten over it. I'm pretty sure.

Chapter Twenty-Seven

GYM CLASS (TAKE IT EASY - WE'LL GET THROUGH IT!)

If recess and lunch are purgatory, gym class is ... well, it ain't heaven.

Some children with autism spectrum disorders are athletically gifted. The rest are usually a little less than devastatingly agile, to put it delicately. My son tends to lumber, rather than walk, and his chosen form of physical exercise is the playing of video games, in which he can assume the shape and dexterity of an over-trained athlete without ever having to break a sweat. He has the most fully developed thumb muscles in the neighborhood.

Even those who are blessed with athletic bodies and the willingness and ability to use them, if they have a spectrum disorder, tend to gravitate toward individual sports like tennis or golf, rather than team sports like baseball or basketball, because they require less interaction with peers, and rely entirely on the ability and determination of one person. Great dedication can pay off, and you never have to worry about someone else on your team forgetting the rules or making an error – a relief for many on the spectrum.

So imagine the joys of gym class, the place where everyone, regardless of race, creed, or athletic ability, is required to participate in sports, and to do so in front of their classmates. For a child with an autism spectrum disorder, this is a perfect storm of embarrassment, setting the child up for failure in more ways than one book could possibly encompass.

Begin with the fact that virtually every activity in gym class can be classified as a team sport. That means the child is required to cooperate with others, no matter who the "others" may be, follow rules whether the others are doing so or not, and perform up to the standards the other children in class would expect, or have the whole team fail as a result.

Character building? It could be seen that way, I suppose. Another interpretation would be that this scenario takes every anxiety most children with spectrum disorders have, blends them together, and concentrates them into one 45-minute period that the child must face every school day.

It's not surprising that so many children with autism spectrum disorders dread gym class even more than we did when we were in school. It's not surprising, either, that some parents of children with spectrum disorders try hard to ensure that their children never have to do so.

Even in school districts that, as most do, require physical education as part of the daily schedule because they are mandated to do so, some parents whose children have autism spectrum disorders have requested – and in some cases received – accommodations that are written into IEPs, excusing the child from participating in gym class. Period. When the parent can demonstrate that the class is harming the child, that his disorder is making it impossible for him to participate without doing himself damage (particularly in social skills, which is the top priority for many children with spectrum disorders), some school districts have made an exception and kept children out of physical education entirely.

The question here is not so much whether your school district will do as you ask, but whether it's a good idea to ask for it.

An argument may be made for having a child with a spectrum disorder skip gym class. It does nothing to help her social development, and in many cases does everything to work against such development. It works against the child's nature in almost every way imaginable. In some schools, it requires changing clothes and showering after class, in a group – something that many of our children find intolerable. And, to be fair, in many cases, the children aren't getting anything out of the class.

On the other hand, there is a strong argument – perhaps just as strong – to be made against the idea. In my son's case, I know that gym class is pretty much the only time during the average day he's going to be doing anything resembling exercise. This is helpful to his overall health and, to a lesser extent, to his understanding that exercise is an important part of a daily routine.

Also, it forces him to interact with other kids, even if he's not happy about it. Teamwork will be required in almost any profession he might eventually choose to pursue, and he will have to learn to do it some time, even with people he doesn't necessarily like. It's not an easy concept, and not a fun one, but a necessary one, and school is the best place for children to learn something like that, isn't it?

I'm not here to tell you what's best for your child; in many cases, the experience of going into gym class every day is more than a child with an autism spectrum disorder can handle. But in my experience, and that of my son, I can say that making "an example" of him by removing him from gym class would have done more to diminish his self-esteem than being relieved of the responsibility to play basketball for one school period a day would have done to build it.

Josh does not look forward to gym class, and he never has. The other children were guaranteed to be "cheating" as he saw it, and that failure to follow the rules as they were explained to the class was often more than Joshua could tolerate. Almost all of the difficult "incidents" he's had in his 11 years of attending school have been at recess, lunch or gym class. I can't remember one that ever happened during math, for example.

At one IEP meeting, it was suggested, just as an idea, that it was not entirely necessary for him to attend gym, that he could be assigned a study hall by himself or a "free period" with his aide, Mrs. Gregus. But after a short discussion, that idea was shelved by everyone in the room, including the person who had brought it up, as the wrong thing for Josh. He would have hated feeling that "different," and having everyone in class know he was "different," more than he hated the games about which he was constantly complaining.

One parent in Kentucky told me that her son had refused to go to gym after making mistakes that he felt had cost his team a game during gym class. His mother suggested that he go to class the next day and pay close attention to the other children and what they said to him. He reluctantly agreed, and came home the next day to report, somewhat sheepishly, that everyone in class had forgotten about his poor performance – except him.

Another mom, however, told me that her son, growing up in Oregon, had finally been removed from gym class, but not because of inappropriate behavior by the other children in his class, or because he was being disruptive when the games didn't go his way.

"The teacher was constantly telling him that he was no good, that he never would be any good, and that everyone was laughing at him," she says. "I didn't see any way to deal with it other than to get (my son) out of that class – there wasn't another gym teacher in the school."

We had one encounter in primary school with a gym teacher in whose class Joshua was apparently being a problem. Josh was coming home telling us that the gym teacher "didn't like him," and was always yelling at him. When we met her at Back to

School Night, the teacher said there had been problems, but she was handling them.

My wife and I were seriously inexperienced at dealing with schools at that point (I think Josh was in first grade), and decided that if the teacher said she was handling it, she was handling it. Besides, what possible problem could be that serious in first-grade gym?

The problem went on for a while, until Josh said he wouldn't go to gym class any more, and one day, after a heated debate with the teacher, he stormed out of the gymnasium during class. The teacher, charged with watching 26 six-year-olds, couldn't leave the room, but called down to the school office to alert the principal.

He, a very calm and sensitive man who was as good an administrator for small children as I've ever met, left his office immediately, and caught a glimpse of Josh walking toward the door of the school. In order to see what Josh would do, the principal made sure he wasn't in Joshua's line of sight. He said later that Josh marched to the door, then seemed to think about what would happen if he left, and hesitated.

At that point, the principal walked over to my son and they discussed the problem. It was decided that we needed to talk to the gym teacher, and Josh would stay out of gym class for the rest of that day, until a meeting could be scheduled.

My wife and I did go in to see the gym teacher, whom we had by now decided really did dislike our son. We had built up a head of steam by the time we got to school that night. We started the discussion by asking what had set off the disagreement that had sent our son to the brink of trying to leave the building and walk his 7-year-old self home, a mile across town.

"It's the same thing as always," the teacher answered, seemingly surprised. "Didn't he tell you?"

We admitted that Josh had been too upset to talk about the cause of the incident, but decided to leave out the part about how the teacher "hated him," thinking that might be a little overstated.

"It's his shoes. He wears sneakers with laces, and he doesn't tie them well enough yet, so they keep coming undone. I'm afraid he's going to trip over them and hurt himself."

That was the problem? The teacher assured us it was.

"We'll get him a pair of shoes with velcro closure," my wife promptly said.

The gym teacher was amazed that we'd agree to do something so simple just to make peace in her class. We bought Josh a new pair of sneakers without laces just to wear to school, and had him practice tying his laces at home. Things calmed down in class to the point that Josh actually seemed to enjoy it for a couple of days.

And that teacher became our strongest advocate in school, always standing up for Josh when he needed defending, and attending our IEP meetings to see if she could help.

If we'd simply taken him out of gym class, we would never have found that advocate, and he would have been prevented from making a friend.

You never know how things are going to work out. If your child is so troubled by gym class that it has become a detriment to his education and his social development, removing him from class might be the best solution. But my advice would be to exhaust every possible answer that keeps him in class before taking that step, because it's a tough one to reverse with our children – once they establish a new routine, going back to the old one can be awfully difficult.

"I hate to take a child out of class for good," one teacher in New York told me. "I don't like the precedent it sets, and I don't think it does the student any good."

After all, it might all just be about the shoes.

Chapter Twenty-Eight

MIDDLE SCHOOL

Every year, we'd hear the same thing from friends and relatives whose children were just a little bit older than Josh: "Next year," they'd say, "is when things really get rough."

It didn't matter that they'd told us this the year before, and the year before that. The following school year, we were assured each June, would be the one that would try our son to his limits and us to the point of despair. "Brace yourselves," they'd say, "the storm is coming this time."

Each year (after the first one), we'd smile and nod, and agree, yes, the coming school term would no doubt be a minefield of difficulty. And my wife and I would exchange a look that said, yeah, sure.

What got our attention was when Joshua's teachers, at the end of his sixth-grade term, took us aside and said, "You know, middle school is a lot different. It's not going to be easy for Josh."

When you hear it from a teacher, it's different. This time, we were concerned.

For neurotypical children, the middle school years (generally speaking, sixth to eighth grade) are no picnic, and for children with disorders on the autism spectrum, you can multiply difficulty in many situations by a power of two. So if we remembered our middle school years (when they were called "junior high school") with a certain degree of dread, we could only imagine what it be like for our son and his Asperger Syndrome.

Having survived those years, I am here to tell you that it's really not all that bad. Did other kids get on Josh's back, when they hadn't before, about his stimming (which has decreased in intensity) and his "unique" turn of phrase? Certainly. Was the schoolwork more challenging in a number of subjects? Sure. Did the change to a new, larger building, requiring faster class changes and a new room for every subject, test Josh's organizational skills, which weren't exactly stellar to begin with? Absolutely.

Was it hell? No. It was school, on weak steroids.

Middle school is the time when those demon hormones start kicking in with students. This is when many children define their roles within the group, and for a good number of children with autism spectrum disorders, that role becomes "the weird kid," something no parent on earth would wish for a child.

Cliques form, alliances change, friends abandon friends with no clear provocation. In middle school, sometimes called the cruelest years a child spends in school, socialization becomes more important than it ever has been before, and that is not good news for a good percentage of our children.

So don't mistake what I'm saying: Middle school is difficult, more difficult, probably, than any years that precede it, but it's not the horror show you might be led to believe. In some ways, middle school was easier for Josh than elementary school, because he wasn't dependent on one teacher for every subject. If that one teacher doesn't grasp the subtleties of your child's disorder, the entire school day can be a trying experience for your child. In middle school, where the teacher changes with each subject, one teacher who doesn't "get" autism and related disorders is only one part of a much larger picture, and sometimes can be more easily overlooked, or the child can be moved to another class with considerably less angst than in a lower grade.

Changing classes is probably the most challenging part of the new experience for children with an autism spectrum disorder. It requires a good number of skills they find difficult to summon, and increases their level of frustration; never a good thing. Moving from room to room in a specified number of minutes (usually not many) also adds to stress, as our children tend to be a little less organized than most, and at the same time a little more concerned about following the rules and showing up on time.

So the stress level increases between elementary school and the first year of middle school. In Josh's case, his aide, Mrs. Gregus, helped him through the more difficult organizational parts, especially those involving finding the room where the next class was held. But within a week or two, he had the lay of the land down and could navigate the school well on his own.

The schoolwork was a little more difficult, but that is true in each successive school term, so that wasn't a big surprise, nor a huge problem. The real academic questions would be raised when Josh began high school, but that's a subject for another chapter.

Social skills play a considerably different role in middle school than in earlier grades. Where kindergarten children might be using their social skills simply to identify themselves to each other, and to find out who the other children are, middle school students are concentrating less on individual identity (at least, outwardly) and more on being part of the group. And that means identifying a group the student wants to join – and eventually finding out if the group will accept a given student. A good deal of self-esteem is on the line, and for students with autism spectrum disorders, there isn't always a happy ending.

If there's one thing we each remember about our experience in the pre-teen and early teen years, it is an obsession with being "cool." Being considered outside the group, outside the (if you can pardon the expression) mainstream, and in some way "flawed," was the ultimate humiliation. It was like being thrown out of the cave and left to deal with the ferocious animals on our own. Being cool, whether in the James Bond mode I grew up with or the hip-hop style that might be the touchstone today, was what it was all about. And to be considered "uncool" was to belong nowhere and be nothing.

Little has changed in the "cool" department, except the pop culture icons by which one's cool quotient is measured. In middle school, it's still all about being in or out, accepted or not, cool or ... not. For students with spectrum disorders, it's harder to be cool than for most everyone else.

Think about it: The ultimate in cool is to be more grown-up, to be unaffected by difficult situations, to be wanted and popular with the group. For most of our children with spectrum disorders, the emotional maturity level is noticeably lower than their chronological age. They are less likely to handle difficult situations unemotionally, and might exhibit more emotion than is appropriate for many situations, because they're not sure where the line is drawn between seeming like they don't care and seeming like they care far too much. Their interests might not coincide with those of their peers, either – Josh probably can't name three artists with popular songs at the top of the charts right now, because he doesn't care, and rarely listens to music. Ask him who designed the hot video game, however, and he can give you all the background and probably point out ways the game could have been made better.

As for popularity within the group, students who don't dress with an eye toward everyone else's taste, who pay no attention to the latest trends in ... anything, who can't be counted on to react with an age-appropriate response to any given situation, will probably not be at the top of the popularity charts. Add to that the difficulty many of our children have in athletics and you have a recipe for, if not disaster, certainly something less than raving success.

Unfortunately, there isn't much we can do to increase our children's popularity with peers. We can make sure the other students understand about autism and related disorders; we can show them videos and have doctors and others lecture to them, and that can make a difference in some cases. But it's not going to make our kids "cool."

What we can do is pay attention to those areas that some children on the spectrum do not notice. We can see what the other students are wearing, and even if we might find the fashions less than appealing, we can see to it that our children look like they fit in. We can strike up conversations with our children about current topics, see what they know and don't know, ask them questions about what other students are discussing and see if they have an idea. If our children have an interest in an area that other students their age might find appealing, we can encourage our kids to pursue that interest.

My wife and I might be the only parents in America to have bought their son a video game system because they thought it would be good for him. When Josh was not yet in middle school (he was probably about 8 or 9 years old), and after a good deal of discussion, we bought a used Sega Genesis system in the hopes that it would give him something to talk about to other children his age, since he seemed to be having a good deal of trouble finding topics to discuss, and was retreating into himself.

It worked far beyond our expectations – probably more than we wanted it to. Within months, Josh was asking for a new system with better games, and after a while, a Nintendo system replaced the old Sega. Since then, PlayStation and then its cousin, PlayStation 2, have displaced the Nintendo, a GameCube has joined it, and he's still hoping for more and better systems, which is one reason we're encouraging Josh to find himself a part-time job.

But his social position changed as well. Suddenly, Josh could discuss the merits and limitations of each game with other children at school, and they would respond. He could invite friends over to play video games (there is one downstairs with him as I type this), and as he became more interested, his knowledge of the video game scene, fueled by magazines and television programs, became prodigious. Other students discovered they could ask Josh for information about games, and he almost always had the answer.

I'm not saying that video games made my son the most popular kid in his class, or even that it made him popular at all. I wouldn't argue for one moment that his time spent playing video games shouldn't be decreased to make room for reading and physical exercise, but I can say without any hesitation that he has a few friends because of the decision we made to introduce him to games.

That's a big step, and in middle school, having an interest that gibes with that of others in the class is a huge advantage. Being able to hold his own in a discussion of a topic other kids found relevant went a long way toward getting Josh out of the area where people who are teased live, and into the one where at least the other students know his name and understand that he can be a valuable person to know.

Middle school isn't the worst thing that can happen to your child with a spectrum disorder. It is a time when things are difficult, but can be managed. It is a place where some skills that will be necessary for life will be learned. It is a time of life when there are still endless possibilities, and students can begin to explore them.

And if all else fails, keep in mind that middle school, at most, only lasts three years. It's the shortest step in a school career, and there's a reason for that.

Chapter Twenty-Nine

TRANSITION

There's nothing on this planet like high school. Except middle school.

All the concepts that went into the discussion of middle school in the previous chapter apply to the high school years, but thankfully, some of the difficulties actually begin to ease when your child becomes your teenager.

Of course, all the difficulties of being a teenager start to kick in right around then, so it's your call whether this is a bargain or not.

The way most adults talk about high school as a viper's nest of cliques to which they were not admitted, hormones they could not keep under control, teachers who were one step short of Fascists, parents who believed *Leave It to Beaver* was real and academics that would put the graduating class at Harvard into a tailspin, it's a wonder anyone ever willingly attends a high school reunion. Who would want to relive all that?

Well, the truth is, maybe it's not as bad as we portray it. Maybe our memories are a little changed by time. Maybe what we're remembering is just the really intense day we had here or there during four years of learning to be a little bit more like adults, and we weren't really in the constant agony we seem to recall.

Of course, the part about the hormones is true.

For a teenager with an autism spectrum disorder, high school presents the same challenges that middle school did, but the teasing might be a bit less intense. Psychologists tell us that high school-age students are more reasonable than those of middle school age, that the cliques and the humiliation aren't as intense in high school, and that students who are "different" are more apt to be accepted, or at worst, ignored during the four-year ramp-up to college or "the real world." And since they're psychologists and we're not, we'll have to take them at their word, for the time being at least.

The one thing I can report after one year of the High School Chronicles for my son is that the academics are more complex, but not so much that students who have been doing well up to this point suddenly begin to fail miserably. Josh has had some bumps in the road along the way, but for the most part, the transition to high school was about the same as the transition to middle school, and maybe a little bit easier.

In some cases, moving from a neighborhood elementary school to a regional middle or high school can be a huge problem for a student with a spectrum disorder. Suddenly, the other students who have known your child for years and have grown used to his "quirks" are replaced, or at least many more unfamiliar students will be added to your child's grade, most of whom do not know about autism spectrum disorders, probably don't care, and are on the lookout for someone to humiliate.

Social skills training that hopefully began when your child was diagnosed comes into play very seriously at this point. We, I feel compelled to report, managed to dodge this particular bullet by living in a school district small enough so that all the district's children are in the same school at the same age. Primary school children all went to kindergarten through second grade together, then moved on to the elementary school at the same time, the middle school after sixth grade, and the high school at ninth grade. Very few new students have appeared who had to "get used" to Josh, and certainly, a huge influx of new students did not show up at the same time when he moved from one building to another.

My wife attended a presentation in one of Joshua's classes

when he was about 10 years old, and watched with some rising discomfort as he sat in the back of the room, stimming madly, humming to himself, lost in an Asperger state of mind that had nothing to do with what was going on in the classroom. But she noticed that the girl sitting next to him, who had known Josh since first grade, simply leaned over and grabbed one of his hands. "Josh," she said, "cut it out." Josh immediately stopped his gyrations and focused his attention on the presentation.

If the girl hadn't known him for those years, would she have handled the situation so calmly? Probably not. So while I recommend moving to a district that has this type of system, I can't guarantee you can find one. So let's see what else can be done.

First of all, start discussing any transition, from elementary school to middle school, middle school to high school, and so on, with the Child Study Team members years before the transition actually happens. Find out from parents whose children are a year or two older than yours what the problems have been, but consult with the teachers and team members as well. Ask what their experience has been with children who have spectrum disorders. Apply that to your own child's personality, and see if it has any relevance.

The high school years are especially important if you expect your child to apply to college, because the grades begin to count once your teenager enters the ninth grade and begins to accumulate a grade point average. Academics are important now, and your son or daughter's strengths and weaknesses will be emphasized. Evaluate them yourself, but talk to teachers and administrators about how they see your child doing academically. If tutors will be necessary, begin tutoring as early as possible to avoid embarrassment for your child and to get the most help before a problem shows itself.

From a social standpoint, the situation might be a little better, but it's never going to be perfect. High school is still a collection of groups masquerading as one large group, and in some cases, our children have trouble fitting into any of the subsets.

For Josh, the turning point came when his English teacher, who also directs the school plays, announced open auditions for the first musical of the season. Josh wasn't interested in appearing on stage, but he did find a way to become involved when one of his friends was cast in the play: He would participate in stage crew, building sets and moving props on and off the stage during performances.

To be fair, he had to be coaxed into participating, but once he began, Josh enjoyed helping to construct sets, and he enjoyed the camaraderie of the stage crew, all dressing in dark colors to avoid being seen on stage, and moving large pieces of scenery in and out to accommodate the actors.

By the spring of his freshman year, Josh was performing on stage and directing himself and two friends in recreating an Abbott and Costello sketch (and he has asked me to make it clear that it was not "Who's on First?" because "that's been done to death"). Next year, he's taking theatre arts as an elective.

It was hard to understand why a teenager who had always found it difficult to make friends and sometimes seemed indifferent to his peers would suddenly revel in a collective activity like a stage play, even if working behind the scenes. But the first time I picked Josh up from a stage crew construction session, I realized why this was the thing for him.

It was Asperger Central in the school auditorium that day. I walked in and saw more stimming and less eye contact than in any other place I'd ever been, but they were getting along, accomplishing a common task and even enjoying a few "in-jokes" as they went on. Josh didn't make any lasting friends on the crew, but he didn't hesitate to get involved the next time there was an open call.

Finding a peer group – even if it's a peer group made up

entirely of kids with spectrum disorders – is a huge step for a teenager with social skills issues. And when Josh felt that he fit in with the group, it made all the difference.

A few months after the stage crew experience, Josh told me he was interested in working on the school's video "news report," the 5-minute program put on closed-circuit television for the school first thing in the morning. Since he'd never shown any interest in television (except to watch it) or news (in any capacity) before, his remark made me curious. He explained what his intention was: To become the high school's film critic.

Josh has always been a movie kid: He talks about upcoming movies all the time and can rarely stand to miss a weekend in the dark, waiting for the next movie to be the one he can tell his friends about. So being a film critic for the school fit his personality perfectly, but I wasn't sure the school's television production teacher would warm to the idea. I began to gear up for a possible Guns A' Blazing moment, but it never came.

The teacher, helpfully prompted by Josh's aide, agreed immediately to give the movie review segment a try, and Josh worked very hard getting ready to deliver his first review. He wrote out what he thought was 2 minutes worth of copy to read, then rehearsed it after dinner for us the night before he was to appear on camera.

It ran about 1 minute, if he spoke very slowly.

So Josh, undaunted, went back up to his computer keyboard to work on more words to say, and soon, he had enough to sustain 2 minutes worth of time. He rehearsed it a few more times, and admitted to being a little nervous before going to school the following morning.

By all accounts, the review went just fine, even though it had to be cut to 90 seconds because something else had run over time. Since then, he's been doing two reviews a week, and because the report is sent to every classroom in the school, he's gaining some notoriety. Other students – even upperclassmen – stop Josh in restaurants or at school and talk about the reviews. Even if they don't agree with his opinion, they seem to enjoy the way he expresses it.

That's a huge social step for a student who only a few years ago didn't want his name to appear in an anthology to which he'd donated a poem because "the other kids will make fun of me." And it came as the result of hard work (mostly on Josh's part) and growing maturity (although not growing that fast).

The real trick in high school is to get through it with some self-esteem intact. For those going on to college, or about to enter the work force, transition is the next step, and for many, the last step in a school career.

It ain't easy, but then, what has been so far?

Chapter Thirty

TOMORROW — THE WORLD!

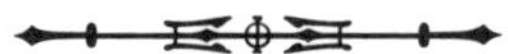

This coming school year, which will start exactly seven weeks from tomorrow, will see my son (about whom you've already heard so much) starting his sophomore year of high school. That means I'm probably already late in starting to plan his transition to college.

With only three years left in the public school system, Josh should already be preparing for life in a larger world, one that at the very least includes driving (!) to class and home every day, and if he's more ambitious, living on campus, or getting a job. We're hoping he'll go to college, but either way, in three years, the public school system will have had enough of him, and send him on his way.

Or will it?

Some transition plans for students who have autism spectrum disorders include the possibility of an extra year in the public school system. During this time the student doesn't attend classes, but works with school personnel on skills necessary to succeed in "the real world," and may work at a part-time job as an element of the extra year program.

For students who have graduated high school, but aren't ready for college or the workplace, this is the equivalent of the transitional primary year between kindergarten and first grade. It's a time when the student is given a chance to "catch up" with the rest of the class, to prepare for the next step and to learn the skills necessary to make that step a successful one.

It's not necessary for everyone, and we're hoping it won't be necessary for our son, but if we see that he's not ready to move on, I'd like to think that I, especially, won't be as resistant to a different idea as I was 10 years ago. Josh has come a very long way since then, but if he still needs extra time, we should see to it that he gets it.

Parents' scariest times of their child's school career are the beginning and the end. When our children start pre-school or kindergarten, we are usually far more petrified than they, and when our children have an autism spectrum disorder, we probably sit by the phone for most of the first week, waiting for what we expect will be the inevitable call to tell us to come and pick up this child and take him home.

But the end of the time at school is more terrifying. We've lived through all the difficulties involved in having a child with a spectrum disorder, the bureaucracy, the bullies, the teachers who don't "get it," the transitions, the tests, the therapies, the social skills training and the tears and laughter. We have navigated waters we once thought were uncrossable. We have watched our children develop from tiny figures intent on getting to snack time into giants, often larger than ourselves, whose thoughts are so complex and personal that we wouldn't understand them if they were expressed to us at all. Which they're not.

We've learned the ins and outs, invented tricks on our own, assessed the personnel and the curriculum, had endless meetings, signed a few IEPs (some of which we actually agreed with), spent countless nights asking and answering questions preparing for tomorrow's quiz or test, called other children's parents for reasons that were either difficult or really difficult, trudged through subject matter we didn't understand when we were in school, applauded the successes, mourned the failures and gotten to know each and every last employee of our district's school system.

And now we're being told that our job is done and that we should step aside for the next guy.

When your child comes of age, and is capable in the law's eyes of making his own decisions, you can huff and puff and blow the school's doors in, but that 18-year-old is an adult in the wisdom of the state, and no matter what you think, if he isn't in some way incompetent, he gets to decide for himself. You wanted it when you were 18, and guess what – he wants it now. And the law says he can have it.

At the IEP meeting we had only a few weeks ago, my wife and I were asked to sign a form that indicated we had been made aware that our son, then 15 years old, would be of age in this state in less than three years, and that he would have the power to make any decisions regarding his welfare after that date. We signed it, because he will.

That's a major reason to begin a transition program years ahead of time. Get your child used to the idea, whether it means a year of working part time under school supervision after graduation, or if it's just a way to get him the information he needs to prepare for the next phase of his life. It's not too early to think about this even in middle school, but the second year of high school, when we're beginning, is about the longest you should wait.

One New York woman told me her son, now 32 years old, was diagnosed at 19, and "never got the right kind of preparation. He had a rough road. Around the age of 23, he started not doing well, making less and less contact with people. Perhaps having all the right kinds of supports along the way would have helped."

Now, she notes, after a rough period, her son's "life is moving nicely. He's such a real person," she adds.

"(My son) never knew what he had," she says. "The children who have early intervention are blessed."

One way to make a smooth transition is to begin it before the traditional moment for the transition, to mix it in carefully and let the student become acclimated to the situation. One New Jersey mom told me her son is attending some college classes before his high school graduation, since the subject matter is more specific to his interests and more challenging to him academically than the routine high school curriculum. Her son will receive a high school diploma upon completing the courses he's taking now. The school district is interested in expanding the program for other students who might benefit from more college-level experience.

Transition from one type of school to another is not easy, but transition from school to adult life is a whole new ballgame. One parent from Pennsylvania told me she "is more nervous about the end of school than any other step along the way." Her son is 9 years old, and she's already worried.

Moving into the work force is a huge step, and rarely an easy one. As Josh approached his 16th birthday, my wife and I were very diligent in suggesting he apply for a part-time job, not only to discover what working is like, but also to fund some of his more expensive habits (video games don't grow on trees).

Surprisingly, our son was open to the suggestion, almost to the point of enthusiasm, which is something of a small miracle in a teenager. He thought for quite some time about what kind of job might be appropriate for him, and after inquiring at all the local video game stores, determined that he might find the best part-time job for himself at an area movie theatre.

He called the theatre, spoke to a manager and asked me to drive him to the theatre to fill out an application. About a week later, the manager called to invite him in for an interview. Josh was noticeably edgy before going in.

"It's an interview for a part-time job," I told him. "It's selling popcorn and cleaning up candy wrappers. Just relax."

"I know," he nodded. "But I've never done this before. What if I give a wrong answer?"

"There's no such thing as a wrong answer," I told him. "The worst thing that can happen is you walk out exactly the same as you are now, and that's not so bad."

I don't know if this advice helped, but Josh seemed more relaxed when the manager, a young woman maybe five years older than he is, appeared to bring him in for the interview. I strolled the mall, waiting for my cell phone to ring.

The interview took only about 15 minutes, and Josh said he thought it went well. When asked why he wanted the job, he told me he responded, "because I love the movies, and I need the money." That seemed reasonable to me.

As it turned out, Josh didn't get the job (he was still 15 years old at the time, and the company requires a minimum age of 16). But he was encouraged to call back after his birthday, and that situation is still pending, since we first want to see how the academic year goes. He's also been savvy enough to fill out applications at other places of employment.

But deciding on an area that interested him was important. Josh might believe the job will be all watching movies at the multiplex, but at least he's already concerned with working at something he likes to do. And now that he's been through the interview process and filled out some job applications, the process no longer seems scary or intimidating.

Personally, my wife and I are just hoping he can pay for his own games.

We hope (and expect) that our son will attend a four-year college after he graduates from high school. He is qualified academically, and high functioning enough that we believe he is capable of handling the transition (we are working on a transition plan with the school district that has not taken clear shape yet). But whether he'll be able to live on campus, as he often says he would like to do, is still very much up in the air.

Going out on their own is something that is daunting for some neurotypical students, and for students with spectrum disorders, it becomes a much more complex issue. Simple lifestyle elements like personal hygiene, interpersonal relationships with other students, laundry, food and navigating the campus are all amplified by a spectrum disorder. It's a lot to try and tackle at once. Add to that the academic workload at virtually any college, and the situation is twice as intimidating.

For Josh, the jury is still out on campus life. For others, the transition has been daunting, and not always successfully handled.

One young woman with an autism spectrum disorder told me that college was a liberating experience after high school, which she found extremely difficult. "I can empathize with a gay kid growing up in a fundamentalist Christian household," she says. "But until I'm that gay kid, I can't know how it feels. In high school, I was afraid to open my mouth, but it got better when I went to college, because I met people who wanted to be animators, like I did, and I could talk to them."

Another, still in high school, is defiant about her autism, does well in classes, and says that since she has been included in mainstream classes, she has not had problems with the attitude of other students. She is applying to colleges now, and says she will live on campus: "There's no reason I shouldn't."

Many colleges and universities are now more aware of autism and related disorders than they were even a few years ago, but they are not inclined to offer accommodations outside counseling, when necessary, and other basics. Laws vary from state to state, but they usually require some sort of transition opportunity. "They're not giving you a break because you're autistic," one guidance counselor told me about colleges. "You're expected to do what the other students do, and if you can't, you can leave, just like them." Colleges and universities are generally sensitive to people with spectrum disorders, and for those who are accepted and who choose to identify themselves as needing accommodations, help is available.

Greg Moorhead, director of disability services for Rutgers University, says that colleges and universities are seeing a much higher number of applicants on the spectrum, particularly with Asperger Syndrome, and that proper accommodations are being made – after the student is accepted.

"The criteria for admission are not changed by a disability," Moorhead says. "The student applies and is accepted or not based on the same things as any other student."

Once the student is accepted for admission, however, he can take the documentation of his disorder, from a clinician or a physician, to the Office of Disability Services, and once that documentation is approved by a committee, the student may request various accommodations, similar to those listed in an IEP.

"Maybe they need quiet settings or extended time for taking exams," Moorhead says. "If everything is approved, the student can go to the disability services coordinator at the beginning of each semester, and they are given a letter for them to deliver to their professors that explains the accommodations that have been approved." Students do not have to apply for the accommodations each semester or each year – they apply as long as the student is active at the university. If new needs arise, there will have to be another application for an accommodation, however.

Moorhead says he is seeing a greatly increased population of students with Asperger Syndrome and other spectrum disorders, and expects that number to climb for the foreseeable future. He is coordinating workshops and programs to help university personnel, particularly in the Student Affairs Office, understand spectrum disorders and what can be done to help students whose difficulties may be less academic and more tied to social situations and campus life.

"They may have difficulty understanding how to relate to classmates of the opposite sex, for example," Moorhead says. "We need to help them understand what is appropriate and what is not appropriate."

In the classroom, it may be possible to develop a contract between the student with a spectrum disorder and the professor to help the student understand the appropriate number of questions that can be asked during a typical class session without overwhelming the rest of the class. Moorehead is exploring that possibility, among others.

Whether going to college or entering the work force, the step out of the school system and into a larger universe is a tricky, and scary, one. But given the incredible resiliency and determination of most people with autism spectrum disorders, there is no reason why it has to be an impossible one. Is it difficult to work with other people, to take supervision, to even get out of the house in the morning and get to work on time? Of course it is, and for those with spectrum disorders, it is even more difficult. The workplace offers all the stress of academia, with added rules that aren't posted or handed out on paper – they're implied, and many of them require social cues. For people with spectrum disorders, this is a new world, and often a very scary one.

But it's not insurmountable, and with a transition plan and proper preparation, it can be a freeing experience. As with everything else involved with spectrum disorders, it requires a lot of preparation.

You've read a lot about my son in this book, maybe more than you care to know. But that's only because my pride in what he has accomplished is a little difficult to contain. And I have no doubt that, upon graduation from high school, he will continue to astonish me with his abilities. I don't take credit for what he has done – they're his accomplishments – but I believe that my wife and I helped pave the way by realizing that school systems aren't expected to be perfect, but they are required to be fair, and by pushing (with the help of many on the other side of the desk who agreed with our philosophy) constantly to see that our son's school was fair to him. Given that amount of leeway, he has done great things, and I expect the best is yet to come.

Your child can do the same. Just keep those weapons holstered unless it's absolutely necessary.

APC

Autism Asperger Publishing Co.
P.O. Box 23173
Shawnee Mission, Kansas 66283-0173
913-897-1004 • www.asperger.net